18 NATURAL WAYS TO BEAT CHRONIC TIREDNESS

Keats Titles of Related Interest

18
NATURAL WAYS TO BEAT CHRONIC TIREDNESS

Norman D. Ford

KEATS PUBLISHING, INC.
NEW CANAAN, CONNECTICUT

18 Natural Ways to Beat Chronic Tiredness is not intended as medical advice. Its intention is solely informational and educational. Please consult a medical or health professional should the need for one be indicated. The information in this book lends itself to self-help. For obvious reasons, the author and publisher cannot take the medical or legal responsibility of having the contents herein considered as a prescription for everyone. Either you, or the physician who examines and treats you, must take the responsibility for the uses made of this book.

18 NATURAL WAYS TO BEAT CHRONIC TIREDNESS
Copyright © 1993 by Norman D. Ford

ISBN 0-87983-612-1

Printed in the United States of America

Keats Publishing, Inc.
27 Pine Street (Box 876)
New Canaan, Connecticut 06840-0876

ACKNOWLEDGMENTS

With a few exceptions, this book is based on documented studies conducted by prominent researchers working at some of America's most distinguished university medical centers. So many sources were drawn on in researching this book that it is impossible to acknowledge them all.

However, I would like to acknowledge my debt to the research carried out by: Robert Hirschfield, M.D., chief of the Mood, Anxiety and Personality Disorders branch at the National Institute of Mental Health and also by the institute's director, Lewis Judd, M.D.; Thomas Roth, M.D., and Timothy Roehrs, M.D., of the Sleep Disorders and Research Center, Henry Ford Hospital, Detroit; David Burns, M.D., psychiatrist, Presbyterian Medical Center, Philadelphia; Gary Holmes, M.D., and the Viral Diseases branch of the Centers for Disease Control, Atlanta; Nelson Gantz, M.D., professor of medicine at the University of Massachusetts Medical Center; Paul J. Rosch, M.D., President, American Institute of Stress, Yonkers, N. Y.; Anthony Komaroff, M.D., chief of the Division of General Medicine, Brigham and Women's Hospital, Boston; John W. Martin, M.D., chief of immuno-pathology, University of Southern California; Michael Pol-

v

lock, Ph.D., director of the Center for Exercise Science, University of Florida, Gainesville; and James M. Rippe, M.D., of the Exercise Physiology and Nutrition Lab, University of Massachusetts.

I would also like to acknowledge the following institutions whose staff made available extensive files and literature on fatigue research: the School of Medicine's Fatigue Clinic at the University of Connecticut; the Sports Psychology Lab, University of Wisconsin, Madison; the National Institute of Allergy and Infectious Diseases; the Stress Reduction and Relaxation Program at the University of Massachusetts Medical Center; and the National Chronic Fatigue Syndrome Association, Kansas City, Missouri.

CONTENTS

vii

Abbreviations Used in this Book

ANS	Autonomic Nervous System
CDC	Centers For Disease Control, Atlanta
CFIDS	Chronic Fatigue Immune Deficiency Syndrome
CFS	Chronic Fatigue Syndrome
FF	Fatigue Fighter technique
mg	milligrams
NIH	National Institutes of Health
SAD	Seasonal Affective Disorder

18 NATURAL WAYS TO BEAT CHRONIC TIREDNESS

CHAPTER ONE

Knock Out Fatigue the Natural Way

Chronic tiredness is the epidemic of the nineties. One in every five people who visits a doctor complains of constant, unremitting weariness and fatigue.

A government study made in 1984 showed that 92 million Americans feel constantly tired and that each year, ten million visit a doctor complaining of chronic weariness and exhaustion. Tens of millions of people in this country consider it normal to feel listless and sluggish while untold millions of others constantly function below par. Yet surveys show that four out of five people who complain of chronic fatigue are entirely free of any diagnosable medical or psychological disorder.

When they excluded the 20 percent of people whose chronic fatigue is due to a medical problem, researchers discovered an amazing fact. They found that, despite their chronic tiredness, the remaining 80 percent possess just as much energy as the average person. The problem is that these people have lost the ability to tap into their energy reserves.

Provided you are free of any actual physical or psychological disorder (or drug side effects), the promise of this book is that you can learn to tap into new, much higher energy levels than you now possess. Drawing on new dimensions from the leading edge of nutrition, exercise physiology, stress management and motivational research, this book presents a tested, whole person program designed to enhance your energy and to dispel fatigue.

The program consists of 18 natural Fatigue Fighter techniques, each designed to help you transform yourself from feeling chronically exhausted to having peak physical and mental energy at all times. Even if you have been fatigued for years, by adopting all or most of these simple techniques, you can swiftly learn to tap your hidden energy and become a high-energy person.

WHAT IS CHRONIC TIREDNESS?

Chicagoan Betty Wilson, a thirty-five-year-old mother of two, described it like this:

"At first, there was this gnawing, overwhelming sense of fatigue. I'd wake up tired and be weary all day. But as time went on, I felt chronically exhausted from morning till night.

"I felt anxious and sad and totally drained. It was all I could do to cook one nutritious meal a week for the kids. My thinking was foggy and I could barely concentrate at work. I'd lost all zest and enthusiasm for life, even for tennis, which I'd always enjoyed.

"By seven o'clock I was so completely wrung out I'd collapse into bed. Yet regardless of how long I slept, I'd wake up more tired than ever."

When her weariness began to disrupt her life, Betty made an appointment to see her doctor. The doctor had heard these symptoms a thousand times before.

"I know it's not just all in your head," the doctor said. "You really do feel deep-down dog-tired all the time. But fatigue itself isn't a disease. No one ever died from it. It's a symptom of an underlying condition that could be as simple as insufficient sleep or poor nutrition. Or it could be as serious as a brain tumor or viral pneumonia."

The doctor explained that chronic tiredness can be a symptom of more than 35 common diseases and disorders, some of which could be life-threatening. To eliminate this possibility, he took a detailed history, then gave Betty a complete physical and ordered a full series of lab tests and screens.

But a week later, Betty learned that all her lab tests were normal.

"I can find nothing wrong," the doctor announced. "Of course, it could be a functional disorder that is difficult to diagnose. But the most likely cause of your fatigue is low-grade depression or anxiety."

The doctor made an appointment for Betty to see a psychiatrist. But after taking a careful history and putting Betty through batteries of psychological tests, the psychiatrist was unable to find anything significantly wrong.

"I've discussed this with your doctor," he told Betty, "and we can find no medical or psychological reason for your tiredness. What you have is chronic fatigue. Once physical and psychological illness or drug side effects have been ruled out, most cases appear to stem from the stress and pressures of modern living. That makes it a lifestyle problem. And there's not much that medical science can do to help."

ENERGY SICKNESS: AN AMERICAN PHENOMENON

Betty's doctor had been right. Chronic tiredness is indeed a symptom, a symptom of America's own sickness: our energy-rich lifestyle. We live in a culture in which it is seldom necessary to exert ourselves physically. We have lost our vitality to the automobile, to mechanization and machines, to television and the VCR.

High technology has speeded up the pace of work to where millions of younger people are forced to labor under tremendous pressure and competition. Workers are overwhelmed by mountains of paperwork and by the monotonous tasks they must face. Brutal competition, buyouts and mergers threaten the job security of millions of Americans while devastating social changes fill our days with energy-sapping stress.

After a long, exhausting commute on the freeway, millions of men and women must juggle their off-hours to fit the demands of two jobs, children, cars, money, sex and social obligations while other millions must face divorce or life as a single parent.

Most people still believe that our energy-powered lifestyle

is the "good life." But the plain truth is that it is destroying the one source of energy we all need most—our own! Despite all our time- and labor-saving appliances, more people are chronically tired in the U.S. than in any other country, including some undeveloped countries with borderline nutrition.

SHOOT DOWN FATIGUE-CAUSING DISEASE

I must stress at this point that the chronic tiredness which is the subject of this book relates to the 80 percent of cases that are *not* caused by diagnosable conditions that can be treated by a physician or psychiatrist. Thus the 18 Fatigue-Fighter techniques that follow should be used only by readers who have already been given medical clearance by a doctor.

If you have symptoms of chronic tiredness, your first step should be to make an appointment with your doctor to screen out any possibility that your fatigue may be caused by a medical condition or a psychological disorder. Fortunately, most diseases and dysfunctions of which fatigue is a symptom can be readily diagnosed and successfully treated by a doctor or psychiatrist.

Included among medical conditions of which relentless fatigue is a symptom is a viral disease known as Chronic Fatigue Syndrome (CFS). Officially, it is known as Chronic Fatigue and Immune Dysfunction Syndrome, or CFIDS.

It's important at this point to have a clear understanding of the difference between the condition known as chronic tiredness and the disease known as Chronic Fatigue Syndrome (CFS). This book is about overcoming chronic

5

tiredness, it is NOT about overcoming Chronic Fatigue Syndrome.

CFS will be discussed in depth in the next chapter. Currently, no medical cure exists. If you do have CFS, I have a few suggestions that may help you obtain more effective medical treatment. And with your doctor's permission, you may find some of the natural Fatigue Fighter techniques in this book useful in restoring your energy and in helping you recover.

Although CFS has received all the publicity, it's well to remember that only 4 percent of people complaining of constant fatigue are actually diagnosed as having Chronic Fatigue Syndrome. Meanwhile, statistics show that 80 percent are suffering from common or garden variety chronic tiredness.

RUNNING ON EMPTY

Chronic tiredness implies lacking sufficient physical energy to live a normal life and not having the zest or drive to do a full day's work plus other activities you'd like to do. It implies feeling so bored, anxious or depressed that you have difficulty in focusing your thoughts or in being able to concentrate on a problem. Sex drive, spontaneity, sense of humor, creativeness and self-esteem are all likely to wane. And, of course, it implies feeling constantly tired and weary and drained of energy.

Yet boredom hardly ranks as an illness and the degree of anxiety or depression associated with chronic tiredness may not be sufficiently intense to justify prescribing antidepressants. Actually, chronic fatigue is a gray area between health and disease. It is a sign that something in the bodymind is off-balance but it is not caused by any medical condition or psychological disorder.

STRESS IS THE UNDERLYING CAUSE OF FATIGUE

Almost invariably, the underlying cause of true chronic tiredness is the unforgiving stress of daily life in an advanced industrial society. Virtually all non-pathological fatigue begins with inappropriate beliefs that cause us to perceive life events as threatening and hostile rather than as friendly and safe. This self-defeating outlook swiftly leads to a mild level of depression and anxiety. We become so concerned with survival that we overcommit ourselves and find we have no time for healthful habits. We eat on the run, have no time to exercise and we go to bed only after all our commitments have been met. Millions of men and women in their twenties and thirties openly boast of how little sleep they get. Yet the majority are suffering from genuine sleep deprivation.

The destructive effects of chronic tiredness swiftly pervade every area of life. While a healthy, high-energy person can handle the pressures of modern living, a fatigued person experiences them as burnout. Tight deadlines, a heavy workload or a tiring commute are frequently complicated by concerns about relationships, debt overload or a rebellious teenager.

Today, there is wide clinical acceptance of unrelieved and unresolved stress as the underlying cause of most chronic tiredness. Mild depression and anxiety soon sap all motiva-

7

tion, leading to a sedentary lifestyle and nutritional deficiencies or excesses. Sleep disturbances are common. And the fatigued person feels constantly bored and loses all ambition and hope for the future. All this creates a vicious circle. Without physical or mental exertion the body's energy mechanisms can begin to atrophy.

USE YOUR ENERGY OR LOSE IT

For example, before you can summon the energy you need to exert yourself, you must first exert yourself. To mobilize the energy to walk fifty yards, you must first exert yourself by walking ten yards. Walk ten yards today and by tomorrow, the body will have mobilized the energy to walk twenty yards plus an extra margin. Walk twenty yards tomorrow and the following day, your body will have mobilized the energy to walk fifty yards.

But the body mobilizes energy only when used. Once chronic tiredness destroys all motivation to walk, and walking becomes boring, the bodymind simply freezes. Hence, the biggest problem in overcoming chronic fatigue is to motivate a person to act.

Obviously, chronic tiredness is not something you can cure with medical treatment or drugs. At best, pharmaceuticals can only temporarily alleviate some symptoms. Unless the condition is disease-related, no drug can permanently cure chronic fatigue. Most doctors are aware of this. They also know that some of our Fatigue Fighter techniques could be more helpful and effective than drugs. But doctors schedule only 10 to 15 minutes with each patient and they're far too busy to encourage lifestyle changes.

8

DRUGS ARE NOT A PANACEA FOR FATIGUE

The physician's task is made more difficult because the typical fatigue victim is frequently unwilling to help herself. As a result, doctors write millions of prescriptions annually for antidepressants and other mood-changing drugs. Certainly, these drugs provide a temporary lift to anyone with depression or anxiety. Unfortunately, they also have a disturbing litany of adverse side effects.

Patients who take mood-changing prescription drugs may experience confusion and disorientation, delirium, difficulty in concentrating, memory loss, dry mouth, difficulty in urinating, blurred vision, increased body temperature, sexual dysfunction, weight gain, very low blood pressure, headaches, an accelerated pulse rate or worsening of glaucoma. The intensity and frequency of these side effects increases with age.

Furthermore, chronic fatigue, drowsiness, depression and anxiety are common side effects of a wide variety of modern drugs prescribed to treat other diseases. And to some extent, almost all drugs are immunosuppressive. In fact, it is the widespread concern about the disturbing side effects of prescription drugs that has renewed interest in nondrug ways to overcome chronic tiredness.

FATIGUE-PROOF YOURSELF

Across the nation, the hazards and low efficacy of drug-focused treatments are promoting a renaissance for alternative health care therapies, a movement which is gaining support from thousands of concerned doctors and specialists.

Working with this philosophy, researchers at major university medical centers have made enormous strides in developing new fatigue-fighting techniques that overcome chronic weariness even when all conventional drug treatment has failed. And while psychiatrists do employ drugs in stubborn cases of depression, the consensus of most is that drugs are inappropriate and that natural, nonmedical therapies are far more effective.

The trouble with drugs is that they treat only a small part of the bodymind, while chronic tiredness is a whole-person problem. Although chronic fatigue has its source in the mind, it swiftly becomes a mindbody phenomenon. Inappropriate beliefs create a self-defeating attitude that results in inability to handle the stress and pressure of modern living. Mild levels of depression and anxiety may then appear.

Since our mind and body work in synergy, these subjective states are swiftly translated into physiological symptoms that drain both mind and body of energy. In this way, chronic tiredness becomes a multiple problem that can be solved only by a whole-person, multifaceted approach.

Today, most of us are so obsessed with hi-tech medicine and drugs that we often have unrealistic expectations of what modern medicine can actually achieve. We tend to forget that there are two sides to medical science. One branch, mainstream medicine, consists primarily of for-profit hospitals, physicians and pharmaceutical manufacturers. During recent decades, mainstream medicine has progressively focused on a reductionist philosophy in which more and more specialists concentrate only on a single organ or disease. This is the very opposite of holistic healing. By employing hi-tech equipment, drugs and surgery, mainstream medicine has achieved a high degree of technical success for certain procedures. But any type of mainstream treatment is likely to be impersonal, unpleasant and expensive. Emphasis is on eliminating symptoms rather than on healing the bodymind.

BOOST YOUR VITALITY WITH WHOLE-PERSON HEALING

Because it treats symptoms rather than zeroing-in on the cause of disease, mainstream medicine is often ineffective in overcoming a whole-person problem like chronic tiredness. The other side of medical science has been far more successful. Consisting primarily of the fields of behavioral and preventive medicine, it approaches healing by using an array of natural therapies that function on all levels of the bodymind. This multilevel approach has earned it the names of holistic medicine or whole-person healing.

Both behavioral and preventive medicine are practiced by M.D.s. But unlike their mainstream colleagues, these doctors prefer to minimize use of pharmaceuticals and surgery and to employ harmless lifestyle changes instead. In recent years, the holistic approach has made such progress that we already know how to revitalize the entire energy system without having to resort to drugs or other mainstream treatment.

The good news is that these same holistic healing techniques are freely available for anyone to use. All 18 of the Fatigue Fighter techniques described in these pages are commonly used in overcoming chronic tiredness by the whole-

11

person approach. Many were originally developed at university medical centers while others are frequently practiced in the fields of behavioral and preventive medicine.

Provided your doctor has given you a clean bill of health, you can practice holistic healing on your own. By using an array of Fatigue Fighter therapies, you can fight chronic tiredness on all levels of the bodymind at once.

THE ENORMOUS HEALING POWER OF ACTIVE THERAPIES

The ability to use these techniques places enormous healing power in your hands. But they are powerful only if you act and use them.

It is important to understand that all therapies are either *passive* or *active*. *Passive* therapies are those in which something is given to you, or done to you, by someone else. You, yourself, do nothing but passively receive them. Among passive therapies are drugs, surgery, massage and herbal medicines prescribed by others. Obviously, some passive therapies can be lifesaving, while others provide useful temporary relief. But a holistic array of more active therapies is usually needed to permanently overcome chronic tiredness.

Active therapies, by contrast, are the core of both behavioral and preventive medicine. Typical active therapies include all attitudinal and cognitive training (such as reprogramming your beliefs), exercise, stretching and breathing methods, upgrading your diet and nutrition, and using relaxation, biofeedback, meditation, aversion therapy and visualization techniques.

Each forces us to take an active role in our own recovery and each encourages us to act to help ourselves. Holistic medicine asks us to take control of our lives and to take responsibility for our own wellness. This book will teach you how to regain control of your health and conquer fatigue once and for all.

ENERGY-BOOSTING STRATEGIES THAT OUTSMART FATIGUE

Designed to provide a complete whole-person solution to chronic tiredness, the 18 Fatigue Fighter techniques in this book combat weariness on all levels. By adopting all 18 techniques, you combine motivational, physical, psychological, sleep, cognitive, emotional, behavioral, stress management, nutritional and diet approaches into a single holistic program. As you begin to practice this smorgasbord of healing steps, you swiftly begin to access your body's latent energy. The result is to revitalize the body's entire energy mechanism. Then, for as long as you continue to make the Fatigue Fighter steps a part of your lifestyle, you should continue to remain a high-energy person.

Naturally, you can adopt only one Fatigue Fighter step at a time. But for best results, you should gradually adopt the entire program. That's because the steps work synergistically. Each step you adopt reinforces the benefits of the steps you are already using. The steps are also "dose-related." Each step increases your energy level. Thus the more steps you are using, the greater the benefit.

Taken together, the 18 Fatigue Fighters effectively replace

13

each of your energy-destroying habits with an energy-building habit. In the process, they should block the constant drain on your energy created by emotional stress. Simultaneously, they should mobilize and conserve your energy, then channel it to power your mind and muscles.

SELF-HELP FOR CHRONIC FATIGUE

This book actually contains 24 Fatigue Fighter techniques, including three methods for boosting motivation, plus at least 50 other action steps to help you defeat chronic tiredness. However, the Fatigue Fighter steps are numbered in such a way as to total 18. The Fatigue Fighters are numbered from #1 to #18 in roughly the order you might consider adopting them. If you prefer, however, you can begin with any one that feels right to you. Whichever step you use first should help you to develop increased energy reserves, while the benefits should spill over into other areas of your life.

For example, if you choose to begin with FF#4 (exercise), not only will your muscles become charged with energy but as you use them to walk, clouds of endorphins will be released in the brain that produce an upbeat feeling of optimism and elation. Studies have shown that for overcoming depression, walking is far superior to drugs.

Wherever you begin, our 18-step program will lead to major improvements in your attitude, outlook, motivation and lifestyle. Your overall health will also improve as your risk of cancer, heart disease, osteoporosis, diabetes and other chronic diseases goes down.

While most of the Fatigue Fighter techniques have been

used with great success, there is, of course, no guarantee that any one step will work for everyone. Research has shown that each method has been successful at least 50 percent of the time.

Naturally, if one technique is not working for you, you should switch to another. Should you experience any ill effects from any technique, cease using it at once.

HOW TO USE THIS BOOK

The key to beating chronic fatigue is to use a holistic or multilevel approach. This means selecting one or more Fatigue Fighter steps from each approach level. Starting with Chapter 5, each chapter focuses on a different approach to beating chronic tiredness.

Chapter 5, *Boost Your Motivation With Behavioral Medicine*, features the motivation-building approach. It includes three Fatigue Fighter steps, each designed to help overcome the lethargy and inertia that accompany chronic fatigue.

Chapter 6, *Don't Take Fatigue Lying Down*, features the physical exercise approach and includes three Fatigue Fighter techniques. Step by step, these methods take you from having barely enough energy to walk to the bathroom to being able to walk effortlessly for mile after mile.

Chapter 7, *How Stimulants Create Chronic Tiredness*, features the addiction-breaking approach and uses three powerful action steps designed to wean you from dependence on caffeine, nicotine and alcohol. All three stimulants are major destroyers of energy.

Chapter 8, *Foods That Fight Fatigue*, features the dietary

15

approach and includes four Fatigue Fighter steps designed to replace low-energy processed foods with high-energy natural foods.

Chapter 9, *Nutrients That Boost Energy*, features the nutritional approach and its single Fatigue Fighter covers the entire range of nutritional deficiencies that contribute to chronic tiredness.

Chapter 10, *Don't Let Poor Sleep Steal Your Energy*, features the somnology approach and uses a total of five Fatigue Fighter techniques to ensure that you are not depriving yourself of sleep, and that you bounce out of bed each morning bursting with energy and zest.

Chapter 11, *How to Tame Energy-Robbing Stress*, features the stress-management approach and uses three important action steps to help you cope with, and eventually eliminate, just about all psychologically-caused chronic fatigue.

Finally, Chapter 12, *Ten Ways to Fatigue-Proof Your Lifestyle*, shows how to put it all together so that you become, and remain, a high-energy person for the rest of your life.

Of course, if you don't smoke or drink coffee or alcohol you can skip Chapter 7. But for best results, you should include all other approaches in your personal game plan. Millions of Americans are depriving themselves of sleep, sound nutrition and exercise, and their energy levels show it.

Whatever overall strategy you choose, we strongly recommend that you include the physical exercise approach and FF#3, 4 and 4A. But it's equally important to fight chronic tiredness on all levels of the bodymind at once.

Since no two readers will have exactly the same problems or priorities, we have avoided offering any planned strategies for overcoming chronic tiredness. Instead, we believe that by reading this book, you will intuitively recognize those Fatigue Fighter steps that you will want to include in your personal game plan. Once you have taken the first step, the abundant energy resources that still lie latent within your body will begin to emerge.

CHAPTER TWO

Are You Tired or Sick?

Before you even think about using any of the Fatigue Fighter techniques in this book, you must first have a complete medical checkup.

If you have experienced ceaseless fatigue for some time and are constantly tired, if you also experience other symptoms, if your fatigue interferes with work and your enjoyment of life, and if none of these symptoms can be explained by lifestyle habits, you should see a doctor without delay. Or if you have been depressed and your mood is becoming progressively darker, you should make an immediate appointment to see a doctor or psychologist. Persistent fatigue should never be ignored in the hope that it will go away.

Although 80 percent of chronic fatigue is due to lifestyle stress, the other 20 percent could be caused by any of a long list of diseases, some of them serious and some life-threatening. Additionally, fatigue is a side effect of many commonly prescribed drugs. Not until your doctor gives you a clean bill of health should you begin any kind of self-therapy.

Besides obtaining medical clearance, you should ask your doctor to give you permission to use each of the Fatigue Fighter techniques that you plan to take up. And you may need your doctor's specific permission to begin a gradually-increasing program of daily walking exercise and to gradually switch over to a diet low in fat and high in fiber.

SCREENING OUT FATIGUE-CAUSING DISEASE

To diagnose the cause of your fatigue, your doctor will need to take a careful history and to order a complete screening lab exam that may include a urinalysis, a kidney screen, tests for endocrine disease and autoimmunity, a liver function and metabolic test and a complete blood count with sedimentation rate. These tests can reveal much about the physical causes of chronic fatigue and they can help your doctor check the functions of your kidneys, liver, metabolism and immune system. The tests could also point to the existence of anemia or certain types of cancer. Depending on his findings, your doctor might then refer you to a psychiatrist, rheumatologist, orthopedist, neurologist or an immunologist.

If that sounds like an overreaction to something as simple as chronic tiredness, remember that your doctor is not testing you for fatigue. No test exists for detecting chronic fatigue. The tests are to detect the possible existence of such serious diseases as cancer, heart disease, diabetes or kidney disease, in each of which fatigue is a symptom.

Although your insurance may cover the entire cost, you may often save time and money by organizing your information so that the entire examination can be handled during a single office visit plus a followup visit. For example, when you describe your symptoms, have them all written down and listed in order of severity. Nothing throws off a diagnosis more than to announce, as you get up to leave, "Oh, by the way. My most severe symptom is frequent headaches."

You may also possibly eliminate some routine testing by learning a few basic facts about fatigue-causing diseases and drugs. The more you know about chronic tiredness, the more you can do to help your doctor arrive at an accurate diagnosis.

Your doctor will probably conduct the examination in a series of five steps. Naturally, we can't predict in which order each step will be reviewed. But the following information should enable you to handle each step in the most helpful way.

•STEP I: Narrowing Down the Possibilities

Most doctors experienced in chronic tiredness will lead off the interview with questions like those below, each designed to reveal whether your fatigue is physical or psychological in origin or is disease-related. Answering these same questions might also help you to understand the cause of your fatigue.

1. Does your fatigue lessen when you exert yourself physically?

2. Do you wake up exhausted, even after hours of sleep?

3. Is chronic tiredness your only symptom?

4. Has your chronic tiredness persisted for a long period without any physical cause being apparent?

In each case, a "yes" answer tends to indicate a psychological or emotional origin. The fatigue is often caused by stress arising from lifestyle problems centering around family, job or debt.

5. Do you experience insomnia or sleep disturbances, or do you sleep for unusually long hours?

A "yes" answer may indicate depression. Many doctors find that depression and other psychological causes of fatigue often respond well to physical exercise.

6. Does fatigue interfere with an activity that you previously enjoyed?

A "yes" answer could help to confirm depression; it could also indicate a medical problem.

7. Do you worry a lot, especially about family, job or financial problems?

8. Do you find it difficult to relax?

9. Do you find life boring or tedious?

10. Are you a workaholic?

Several "yes" answers may indicate a high level of stress.

11. Does your fatigue disappear on weekends or vacations?

A "yes" answer probably indicates job-related stress.

12. Does your fatigue worsen when you perform some physical activity?

13. Did your fatigue first appear suddenly, such as at 3:00 P.M. on April fifteenth?

A "yes" answer to one or both questions may indicate a physical disease, possibly viral in origin.

21

14. Does your fatigue disappear after a good night's sleep?

A "yes" answer may indicate that you are overcommitted to too many activities and that your problem is sleep deprivation.

15. Are you unusually sensitive to cold?

16. Do you experience shortness of breath?

17. Do you tend to put on weight?

18. When you stand up quickly, do you often feel dizzy?

"Yes" answers to most of these questions could indicate that you have anemia or a low thyroid condition. Both conditions thin the blood and keep blood pressure low, causing the brain's oxygen supply to drop when you stand up quickly.

19. Are you usually too tired to exercise?

20. Do you work at a sedentary job?

21. Are you unable to find time to exercise?

22. Do you sleep nine or more hours each night?

23. Do you watch TV for more than 2½ hours each day?

A series of "yes" answers may indicate that your problem is a sedentary lifestyle. Muscles that are weak and unused result in a flabby cardiovascular system which, in turn, fails to supply the body's muscles and cells with sufficient oxygen. Without an adequate supply of oxygen, the muscles cannot burn glucose for energy, a condition that literally sabotages the body's energy mechanisms and that also leads to poor sleep.

24. Do you experience both severe fatigue and unquenchable thirst?

A "yes" answer could well point to diabetes.

25. Is your fatigue accompanied by swollen glands, dizzi-

ness, muscle aches, headache, poor appetite and low-grade fever?

A "yes" answer could point to a viral infection such as hepatitis or mononucleosis or possibly CFS.

26. Is your fatigue accompanied by frequent mood swings, rapid heartbeat, dizziness and a craving for sweets?

A "yes" here could lead your doctor to test for hypoglycemia.

27. Is your fatigue accompanied by unexplained crying fits, feelings of helplessness and hopelessness, and reduced self-esteem?

A "yes" answer may be a tip-off to clinical depression resulting from a chemical imbalance.

28. Is your fatigue accompanied by weight loss, muscle weakness, insomnia, diarrhea, excessive perspiration and rapid heartbeat?

A "yes" answer could indicate hyperthyroidism.

29. Is your fatigue accompanied by chest pains, shortness of breath, heart palpitations or a feeling of panic?

A "yes" answer could indicate heart disease.

While the diagnosis of fatigue remains an inexact science, a series of well chosen questions such as these can help your doctor to quickly narrow down the possibilities.

•STEP 2: Identifying a Fatigue-Causing Disease or Dysfunction

Chronic tiredness may be a symptom of any one (or more) of the following diseases: adrenal gland deficiency (Addison's disease); adult-onset (Type II) diabetes; AIDS; Alzheimer's disease; apnea; cancer (most types); cardiovascular disease; chronic fatigue syndrome; Epstein-Barr virus; fibromyalgia (fibrositis); heavy metal poisoning (such as lead or solvent in bloodstream); hepatitis; hypoglycemia; hyperthyroidism; iron-deficiency anemia; lingering bacteria or virus infection; liver disease; low thyroid condition; Lyme disease; metabolic imbalance; mononucleosis; multiple sclerosis; muscular dystrophy; nervous system dysfunctions; nocturnal myoclonus; overactive adrenals (Cushing's syndrome); Parkinson's disease; premenstrual syndrome; pulmonary diseases such as viral pneumonia; or renal disease. Chronic fatigue may also be caused by clinical depression or by emotional disorders such as severe anxiety or panic attacks.

By taking a careful history, giving a complete physical and ordering lab tests, your doctor can usually eliminate most of the conditions on this list. Any disease that is diagnosed can then be promptly treated.

The following conditions are among the most common fatigue-causing disorders.

Iron-Deficiency Anemia

Iron is essential to formation of hemoglobin, the oxygen-carrying component of red blood cells. A nutritional deficiency of iron swiftly leads to a low blood hemoglobin level and a reduced supply of oxygen to organs, tissues and cells. Inadequate oxygen supplies immediately inhibit the body's energy mechanisms, resulting in physical fatigue, apathy, irritability and shortness of breath.

Iron-deficiency anemia is a common cause of chronic fatigue in women but may also occur in men. Almost invariably it is caused by a loss of blood. Some women lose large amounts of blood with each menstrual cycle and millions of younger women may be deficient in iron. Energy then virtually disappears and anyone with iron-deficiency anemia feels constantly tired, sluggish and totally incapable of strenuous exertion.

If your doctor suspects anemia, he will order a blood count as part of your screening blood panel. The test shows the percentage of blood cells that are red and also the extent of oxygen-carrying capacity in the blood. A blood iron level test may also be ordered. The results will help your doctor diagnose iron-deficiency anemia or, alternatively, you may have the less common hemolytic or pernicious types of anemia. Accompanying tests may also indicate a deficiency of vitamin B-12. Most cases of anemia can now be treated successfully.

Most physicians will also attempt to locate the source of blood loss. If you are pregnant, nursing, menstruating heavily, have recently undergone surgery, or have a bleeding injury, an ulcer or hemorrhoids, the cause is fairly obvious. Otherwise, your doctor may look for internal bleeding in the gastrointestinal tract.

Most cases of simple iron-deficiency anemia can be treated with iron supplements taken together with vitamin C to aid in absorption. The RDA for iron is 18 mg. Never exceed this amount without consulting your physician first. Your doctor may also give you a vitamin B-12 shot, though this therapy is becoming less popular. You should also try to include in your diet such iron-rich foods as dried beans, spinach and dried apricots and peaches.

In view of a recent study in Finland, which linked above-average blood levels of iron with increased risk of heart disease, cancer, diabetes and other chronic diseases, we advise caution in using self-therapy for anemia. If you suspect anemia, you should have your condition diagnosed by a physi-

25

cian and limit iron supplementation to amounts specified by your doctor. Many processed breads, cereals and flours are enriched with iron. For a nonanemic person, a diet high in fortified cereals and red meat could possibly lead to iron overload.

Hypothyroidism—Low Thyroid Condition

Next to anemia, low thyroid condition is the most common physical cause of chronic tiredness. The thyroid, a small endocrine gland in front of the throat, secretes miniscule amounts of a large protein molecule that governs the body's basal metabolism—the rate at which food is transformed into muscle fuel. A sluggish thyroid slows the entire body's metabolism, including the digestive and energy mechanisms, resulting in chronic fatigue. Simultaneously, all surplus calories are stored as fat and body weight increases.

Other symptoms include feeling cold even when most people feel comfortably warm; mild depression; hair loss; and water retention with swollen ankles. Low thyroid condition is common in America, particularly among women.

Most doctors diagnose hypothyroidism from the patient's description of symptoms. A thyroid panel blood test is available but results are easily thrown off by toxins and are considered undependable. However, a more reliable do-it-yourself temperature test can help your doctor confirm his findings.

To use the test, purchase a basal thermometer at a drugstore. Each morning for one week you must take the temperature under your armpit as soon as you awaken. To do this, you must shake down the thermometer the night before and have it ready by the bedside. Women are usually advised to wait until the second or third day of menstruation before beginning. The normal armpit temperature is 97.8–98.2 degrees. If your armpit temperature consistently reads in this range you probably do not have hypothyroidism. However, if your temperature is below 97.8 degrees for three consecutive mornings, and if other symptoms are present, it may well indicate a low thyroid condition. Inadequate oxidization resulting from hypothyroidism causes the armpit temperature to fall below normal.

In some cases, low thyroid condition may be due to an iodine deficiency. But this is unlikely if you add even a pinch or two of iodized salt to your meals each day.

The more usual procedure is for the doctor to prescribe thyroid replacement therapy, which means you will take a thyroid hormone supplement for life. Since thyroid hormone supplement is a natural body substance, it is not a drug. Even so, side effects may occur in the form of heart palpitations or feeling hyped up and nervous. In this case, your doctor should change your prescription to another thyroid hormone or reduce the dosage. Results may take weeks to appear. But once the dose is correctly adjusted, all your original energy and aliveness should return.

Other Common Fatigue-Causing Diseases

Fibromyalgia or fibrositis is another common cause of chronic fatigue as well as joint and muscle pain. The disease, which primarily affects women between 25 and 50, resembles rheumatoid arthritis and may persist for years. Estimates say it is more common than CFS and afflicts more than five million people in America.

Another fairly common fatigue disorder is *acute* infection

27

with the Epstein-Barr virus, the primary cause of mononucleosis. Fortunately, its effects last for only a few weeks. Both diseases have been mistaken for CFS. *Chronic* Epstein-Barr infection, on the other hand, can last for months or years and is considered one of the possible causes of CFS.

Sleep disturbances such as nocturnal myoclonus or apnea may also cause chronic fatigue. Nocturnal myoclonus, or "periodic leg movement," causes a sleeper to jerk or move the legs hundreds of times each night. At each movement, sleep is disturbed. In apnea, which is most common among overweight, middle-aged men, the air passage in the throat becomes blocked every few minutes by flabby tissue. Several hundred blockages can occur each night and at each one, the sleeper is awakened. Surgery and drugs are available to help apnea victims; a mask can also be worn that fits over the nose to prevent throat blockage. A more dependable solution used by holistic M.D.'s is to have the patient lose weight and eliminate alcohol.

•STEP 3: Identifying Drug Side Effects That Cause Chronic Fatigue

Chronic fatigue may manifest as a side effect of each of these classes of prescription drugs: adrenal steroids; antibiotics; anticonvulsants; antihistamines; antihypertensives (except ACE inhibitors); antiParkinsonian medications; antiarrhythmic drugs; arthritis medications; appetite suppressants; asthma medications; barbiturates; beta blockers; cough suppressants; diuretics; epinephrine; gastrointestinal medications; glaucoma medications; insulin; oral contraceptives; pain relievers (especially narcotics); sleeping pills; steroids (cortisone or other corticosteroids); tranquilizers; tricyclic antidepressants; ulcer medications; and certain drugs prescribed for treating alcoholism.

All too often, these and other drugs may also list depression as a possible side effect. Depression is a major cause of inertia, an attitude which effectively blocks the body's energy mechanisms from functioning.

If your doctor finds that your fatigue is a side effect of a prescription drug you are taking, she may be able to change to another drug less likely to induce fatigue. For example, Dr. Frans H. H. Leenan, associate professor of medicine at the University of Ottawa, recently studied the relationship between beta blockers and fatigue at Toronto Western Hospital.

Many people who take beta blockers for high blood pressure are also told to exercise. But they find that the beta blockers often induce fatigue that inhibits their exercising.

Using male subjects aged 24 to 26 riding stationary bicycles, Dr. Leenan found that the nonselective version of beta blockers prevents the muscles from consuming fatty acids for energy, thus restricting potassium from entering the muscles and causing premature fatigue. The result: men taking the nonselective version could pedal only 30 to 40 minutes after taking a beta blocker compared to 60 minutes after taking a selective version.

ARE MAINTENANCE DRUGS REALLY NECESSARY?

We must never forget that most drugs are prescribed to accomplish only what a healthy body can usually do for itself. By adopting the Fatigue Fighters in this book, we may help to restore lost functions to the point where the body-mind takes over once more and drugs are unnecessary.

Millions of cases exist today in which a person has been placed on expensive prescription drugs for life when an upgraded lifestyle could have achieved even greater benefits at no cost. For instance, at least half of all cases of high blood pressure could be restored to normal by a combination of daily walking exercise and a low-fat, high-fiber diet of primarily plant-based foods. Instead, physicians have prescribed maintenance drugs for life. Admittedly, a sizeable proportion of the American public is unwilling to exercise regularly or to adopt an unfamiliar way of eating. Much the same could be said for people placed on lifetime medication for Type II diabetes or to lower cholesterol.

Excluding causes due to actual disease or to genetic abnormalities, literally millions of Americans have been placed on lifetime maintenance drugs for conditions that result from an unhealthy lifestyle. When health-restoring habits are substituted for health-destroying habits, conditions such as hypertension, Type II diabetes and high cholesterol often disappear. And they remain in remission for as long as a health-enhancing lifestyle continues to be followed.

Pharmaceutical manufacturers are well aware of the tremendous profit potential of having large numbers of Americans placed on maintenance drugs for life. Thus doctors are under enormous pressure from pharmaceutical salesmen to prescribe drugs rather than lifestyle changes. The medical profession should be commended for having resisted much of this pressure. Yet millions of Americans themselves prefer to pop a pill rather than adopt healthier habits.

QUESTIONS TO ASK ABOUT DRUGS

If your fatigue is drug-induced, this might be a good time to ask yourself:

Why am I taking this drug?
Is it really necessary and do I really need it?
What would happen if I did not take it?
Could I replace it with healthier lifestyle habits?

Naturally, the idea here is simply to start you thinking about phasing out any drug you do not really need. If you are under medical treatment for any reason at all, or are taking any medication prescribed by a physician, you must obtain your doctor's consent before dropping it. Furthermore, you may have built up a dependency or addiction to the drug that calls for phasing it out under medical supervision. Under no circumstances should you stop taking a prescribed drug without medical approval.

Nor are we trying to discourage you from consulting a doctor or from taking any drug that is really essential. However, try to minimize your intake of non-essential prescription drugs which can inhibit the benefits of many natural therapies. If you must take a drug, ask your doctor to prescribe the minimum effective dose for the shortest possible period of time. As a general rule, try to take as few drugs as possible.

Instead, ask yourself which alternative therapies might be more effective, less costly and free of destructive side effects. For example, millions of people who are taking prescription tranquilizers could achieve greater benefit by using deep breathing, aerobic exercise and natural relaxation techniques—all much safer, more effective and free of cost.

31

If, despite these suggestions, your doctor wants to over-medicate you, trying to solve all your problems with drugs, you may want to seek a second medical opinion. Some physicians will continue to prescribe a drug even when your problem is one for which drugs are not the best answer. Should a side effect appear, they prescribe yet another drug to minimize the side effect—and so on, *ad nauseum*.

It would certainly be wise to seek a second opinion for any decision to manage depression with maintenance drugs. You should always bear in mind that, far from being the best treatment for your condition, drug maintenance may be prescribed as the treatment least likely to provoke a malpractice suit.

So don't expect the average M.D. to try any unconventional or innovative treatment. Most doctors are terrified of litigation or of being considered nonconformist by their peers. The treatment you're likely to be given is the standard treatment that all other area physicians are using. Surveys have shown, however, that if you are affluent and well covered by insurance, you are more likely to be given an expensive treatment that you don't really need.

Obviously, this section is not directed at that small portion of the American public who do need drugs on a short or long-term basis. But if your doctor appears to favor drugs over improved lifestyle habits, you might seriously consider switching to a physician who is more holistically inclined.

•STEP 4: Diagnosing Depression or Anxiety That May Require Treatment

Both fatigue and depression are listed as side effects of three of the ten most frequently-prescribed drugs in America.

Moreover, the *Physician's Desk Reference* lists depression as a recognized side effect of over 310 prescription drugs. More than 25 percent of all drugs may cause mood swings or unwelcome emotional effects. And while most researchers believe that depression causes fatigue, others have suggested that depression is merely a symptom of chronic fatigue.

One thing is certain. People who are depressed, or suffering from severe anxiety, are seven times more likely to experience chronic fatigue. This finding, by the National Center for Health Services Research, emerged from a recent study which concluded that psychological factors were better predictors of chronic fatigue than physical factors.

An essential step in your medical exam is to ensure that you are free of serious depression or anxiety. Most family doctors can treat these conditions but the majority usually refer patients to a psychiatrist or psychologist for further evaluation. These practitioners have standard tests for diagnosing various levels of depression or anxiety.

Clinical depression is a serious emotional syndrome in which a person feels hopeless, helpless, worthless, and pessimistic and may contemplate suicide. All such cases require treatment by a psychologist or psychiatrist. A milder level known as chronic low-grade depression is characterized by low energy levels, fatigue and poor self-esteem.

Treatment may range from antidepressant medication, which can clear up the condition in four to six weeks, to lifestyle reprogramming such as cognitive positivism, exercise and improved diet, each designed to eliminate the cause of depression. Each of these therapies is among the Fatigue Fighters in this book.

Because they save time and effort, powerful antidepressant drugs are often the treatment of choice. However, antidepressants may be effective only when the cause of depression is at least partially biochemical. By altering brain chemistry, antidepressants are frequently successful in making chronic fatigue disappear, but not without a price. Some of their adverse side effects are listed in Chapter 1. Only subjective therapies, such as cognitive positivism and creative visualization, are capable of rooting out the cause of purely psychological depression.

•STEP 5: Eliminate Chronic Fatigue Syndrome

Eliminating the possibility that you may have CFS remains the final step. To obtain an accurate diagnosis: 1) all other possible diseases and disorders must first have been ruled out; and 2) you must have experienced severe chronic fatigue for at least six months.

The first cases of CFS, or as it is also known, Chronic Fatigue Immune Deficiency Syndrome (CFIDS) began to surface in the early 1980s. At first, physicians considered it a phantom or controversial disease that existed mostly in the patient's mind. But in 1988, it was officially recognized by the Centers for Disease Control (CDC). Their "case definition," published in the March 1988 issue of *Annals of Internal Medicine*, remains the best criteria for diagnosing CFS.

According to the CDC, CFS is diagnosed when:

1. Continued, persistent and relapsing fatigue has occurred for a period of at least six months and has been of such severity that a person must reduce daily activities by more than 50 percent.

2. All other possible fatigue-causing conditions have been excluded through a patient history, physical exam and lab tests.

34

3. The patient has manifested at least six of these symptoms: sore throat, sleep disturbances, mild fever, painful lymph nodes, joint pain without redness or swelling, muscle weakness and pain, headaches, and prolonged fatigue after exercise that is not helped by bed rest.

4. The patient has manifested symptoms of neuropsychological complaints such as: excessive irritability, forgetfulness, depression, confusion, and difficulty in concentrating.

"Yuppie Flu"

Although the disease has struck people of all ages and in all walks of life, it has appeared most frequently in educated, career-oriented white women aged 24 to 45. Surveys reveal that the typical victim is an ambitious over-achiever with a stressful occupation and a busy, fast-paced lifestyle. Many victims also report having experienced depression or food allergies prior to getting CFS.

The disease appears most often after a stressful period in life, particularly after a painful divorce.

Like the flu, CFS often begins suddenly, causing researchers to suspect a viral origin. Yet despite intensive study by teams of virologists, immunologists and endocrinologists, the cause of CFS remains murky. It is a complex disease that appears to overstimulate the immune system and to change key neuroendocrine pathways. Thus far, no lab test can detect CFS. Making the disease even more baffling is that most victims appear physically well.

Although symptoms typically last for three to four years, the majority of CFS sufferers begin to show signs of recovery after the eighth month. Approximately 15 to 20 percent are fully recovered after 12 to 18 months. The majority are able to continue working during the disease and to perform light housework. Yet 5 percent are so severely affected that they must give up their jobs and remain at home, possibly for years. Recovery is often gradual with relapses alternating with bouts of improvement. Fortunately, the disease is not fatal.

While pain relievers are often prescribed to relieve aching symptoms, orthodox medicine currently has no standard treatment for CFS. Individual doctors have reported that low doses of antidepressants, sedatives and anti-inflammatory agents have apparently blocked immune system receptors, thus relieving some symptoms. Injections of magnesium sulphate have also been reported beneficial. Other physicians have found that combining a high-carbohydrate diet (see Chapter 8) with a graded program of light rhythmic exercise and stretching has proved quite successful.

Almost all physicians agree that following a wellness lifestyle will speed recovery. Smoking, alcohol or illicit drugs, poor eating habits and inability to handle stress all delay recovery.

The consensus of medical opinion is that those diagnosed as having CFS should avoid any strenuous aerobic exercise and should conserve available energy for essential tasks. But while adequate rest is essential, total bed rest should be avoided if at all possible. Space agency tests have shown that total bed rest can cause more physical deterioration in twenty days than most people experience in twenty years of normal living. Another hazard is that total inactivity can lead to an attitude of general inertia: the less we move, the less we want to move.

Bonafide advice about CFS is available by phoning the CDC's Voice Information Systems at 404-332-4555. The National CFS Association (3521 Broadway, Suite 222, Kansas City MO 64111) recently offered to send a package about rehabilitation and support groups to anyone who enclosed one dollar for postage. Several sources have also recently cautioned the public against hype that may promote unproven and often expensive treatment for CFS. While we believe that some of our Fatigue Fighter techniques might help CFS patients recover, we urge you to use them only in cooperation with your physician.

GOOD NEWS FROM YOUR DOCTOR

Most people who seek answers about fatigue from a physician are given good news. Four out of five learn that they do not have any specific, diagnosable or treatable physical or psychological condition. The cause of their tiredness lies in their lifestyle or in emotional conflicts due to job, relationships or money.

Many are so reassured by this news—their relief is so tremendous—that they feel powerfully motivated to begin adopting the Fatigue Fighter techniques right away.

If, instead, your doctor does detect a disease or emotional disorder, the chances are good that it may be nothing more than iron-deficiency anemia or low thyroid condition. Whatever treatment your doctor suggests is likely to end both the medical problem and your chronic tiredness.

The modern view is that orthodox medical treatment can be part of the whole-person approach to healing. Should you require further medical treatment, you can continue to practice the holistic approach by accepting your doctor as a partner while you work together as a team. In this way, you can continue to play an active role in your own recovery.

Obviously, not all doctors fit into this perception. And not

37

all doctors are equally competent. Even within medicine, a second doctor may know of a less expensive, more effective treatment with fewer side effects of which your present doctor is unaware. It's a good rule to avoid any physician who smokes or does not follow the wellness lifestyle, or who is not fit and cheerful and aware that drugs and surgery may not always be the best solution.

A final word about the Fatigue Fighter techniques. While each is considered safe and effective, different techniques, foods or supplements may have varying effects on different individuals. Thus you should have your doctor's consent before undertaking any of the Fatigue Fighter methods in this book.

Assuming that you now have obtained this consent, and that your doctor has also given you medical clearance, you are free to begin practicing each of the Fatigue Fighter techniques in this book . . . and to overcome chronic tiredness the natural way.

CHAPTER THREE

Start Rebuilding Your Energy Now

H ere are ten simple steps to help you begin phasing out chronic tiredness while you are reading the rest of this book. But first, there are two important caveats:

One: since know-how is the key to permanently overcoming chronic tiredness, you must read and absorb the remainder of this book right through to the end.

Two: you must already have been given medical clearance by your physician. The ten action-steps below (and all others in this book) are for use only after your doctor has determined that your chronic fatigue is not caused by any disease or dysfunction, and that these steps are safe for you to use.

TEN SIMPLE ACTION STEPS TO HELP YOU BEGIN PHASING OUT CHRONIC FATIGUE

1. Assuming you are able, walk as far as you comfortably can without becoming tired or exhausted. Stay close to home and take frequent rests if necessary. Take one walk every other day and increase the distance as your energy returns. Alternatively, you could swim or pedal a stationary bicycle.

2. Starting today, cut out 50 percent of all the fat and oils in your diet.

3. Cut your intake of meat, whole milk dairy foods (including ice cream), eggs, fish and poultry in half and replace them with fresh fruits, vegetables, whole grains and legumes (beans).

4. Include plenty of tubers in your diet: sweet potatoes, potatoes, carrots, parsnips, turnips and rutabagas, and also squash. Do not add cream or oil, butter or margarine while cooking. Use only nonfat dressings such as plain, nonfat yogurt.

5. If you usually wake up tired, watch one hour less of TV each night and go to bed one hour earlier. Get up at the same time every morning of the week. Get an adequate amount of sleep each night and do not sleep in on weekends.

6. Reduce coffee intake to a maximum of two five-ounce cups per day.

7. Cut consumption of sugar and all other sweeteners in half. That includes honey and molasses. Cut out candy entirely.

8. Eat only whole grains. Replace any breakfast cereal containing sugar with a healthful whole grain cereal such as shredded wheat or oatmeal. Avoid any bread or baked goods

40

which list "flour," "wheat flour," "enriched flour" or "unbleached flour" ahead of whole grain flours. Eat only breads made exclusively of whole or sprouted grains (often available only in health food stores).

9. Make breakfast your largest meal of the day, followed by a moderate-sized lunch and a light dinner. If breakfast is a rush in your home, the night before prepare a large bowl of cold, whole grain cereal mixed with several chopped fresh fruits (bananas, apples, etc.), and topped with plain, nonfat yogurt. Keep overnight in the refrigerator.

10. For between-meal snacks, eat whole grain bread with sliced fruits, sunflower seeds mixed with raisins, plain air-popped popcorn, rice cakes, or a baked potato or yam.

These steps will get you started. But it usually takes a whole-person approach to permanently overcome chronic tiredness. To learn how to transform yourself into a high-energy person, you must read and absorb the remainder of this book.

CHAPTER FOUR

Everything You Ever Wanted to Know About Chronic Tiredness—But Were Too Weary to Ask

You can swiftly gain power and mastery over chronic tiredness by learning everything there is to know about it. We're not talking about a little knowledge. Incomplete knowledge can be dangerous. We mean learning as much about chronic tiredness as your doctor may know, and possibly more. In other words, we mean becoming a medically-informed layperson—at least, where chronic fatigue is concerned.

This chapter presents an overview of the entire bodymind energy process. Each following chapter then expands on a single aspect of the energy process, while each Fatigue Fighter technique adds more to your knowledge of chronic tiredness and how it occurs. Thus to be completely informed you must read this entire book completely through to the end.

A basic principle of holistic healing is that most diseases and disorders begin in the mind. The mind then transforms psychological abnormalities into physical dysfunctions.

THE MOST COMMON FATIGUE-PROMOTING BELIEF

Vic Smart had always felt tired. When his fatigue and mood swings began to affect his job performance and home life, his wife persuaded Vic to see a doctor. But his physician found no sign of any physical or psychological disease.

"What you have is chronic fatigue, and the best treatment is a regular daily walking program," the doctor advised. "Exercise will revitalize your energy and elevate your mood. Start with half a mile and gradually work up to a brisk three miles each day."

Vic looked alarmed.

"That's work," he exclaimed. "In our family, we've always viewed exercise as punishment."

"Besides," Vic went on, "I don't have the energy to walk

43

even a hundred yards, let alone half a mile. I have no energy at all. I'll never be able to exercise. And there's never any time for walking, anyway."

To the doctor, Vic's abhorrence of exercise sounded like a psychological problem. So he referred Vic to a psychologist.

It didn't take the psychologist long to discover that these same self-defeating beliefs—programmed into Vic from his earliest days—were largely responsible for his chronic tiredness. Vic's grandfather, an old-time farmer who worked his muscles hard all day, had always told Vic that no one needed to exercise. The grandfather equated exercise with work and called it punishment.

A belief like that seemed sound to someone who worked all day with pitchfork and shovel and walked several miles around the farm. Additional exercise didn't sound like fun. But when applied to Vic, who sat in an office all day, it became a self-defeating legacy.

What we believe is what we get!

The belief that exercise is work, and should be equated with punishment—widely held by tens of millions of Americans today—is probably responsible for more chronic tiredness than any other single factor.

HEALTH-WRECKING BELIEFS

Beliefs that may have once seemed appropriate may be draining our energy today. All too often, we grow up conditioned by our parents, teachers or peers to perceive the world through a filter of negative, fear-based beliefs. Instead of seeing a friendly, safe world we may perceive the world as hostile and threatening.

Or, as in Vic's case, negative beliefs may lower your self esteem and set you up for a permanent downer that constantly drains away vital energy.

Almost always, chronic tiredness begins in the mind with a set of self-defeating, inappropriate beliefs. When we perceive the world through a filter of such negative beliefs, we begin to think negative thoughts.

As we think, so we feel.

Thus we begin to experience negative feelings such as fear, anxiety, resentment, anger and unforgiveness. Prolonged exposure to negative feelings eventually leads to such recognized psychological disorders as depression or anxiety.

Most of us are aware that, whenever we perceive something as threatening, we automatically set off the body's fight or flight response. This is a hair-trigger arousal mechanism that prepares the body to meet imminent physical danger. Back in the days of sabre-toothed tigers, the fight or flight response served us well. In a split second, it prepared us to either fight off a threatening enemy or to take flight and flee.

However, most people don't realize that almost any negative emotion can trigger the fight or flight response. The sight of a letter from the IRS may set off the same alarm response as being confronted by a masked gunman. Directly or indirectly, whatever we perceive as negative or unfriendly can put us into an emergency state.

BELIEFS THAT SAP YOUR VIGOR AND VITALITY

For example, a person with a negative belief such as "Exercise is work," can perceive the advice to exercise as a threat.

45

When this happens, in a brief instant the body enters into an emergency state with all systems GO. The response begins when the adrenal glands squirt adrenalin and other stress hormones into the bloodstream to arouse the body.

Breathing becomes rapid and shallow as heart and lungs labor to pump more oxygen-laden blood to energize the muscles. Meanwhile, nonessential activities like digestion shut down and the body's blood-clotting mechanism is activated to prevent bleeding should a wound occur.

Faced with a threat in primitive times, we usually had to act. We either fought or fled and the physical activity released our tensed muscles and our keyed-up crisis state. After the crisis was over, our entire bodymind was relaxed and calm once more.

In modern society, it's not always so easy. Seldom can we defuse the tension by punching an opponent or by running away. Instead, we're forced to stand and listen to the boss's criticism or to the complaints of an angry customer. Instead of being released by exercise, we remain in a lingering alarm state with our muscles still tensed and we continue to feel uptight and uncomfortable.

When the fight or flight state fails to shut off after a perceived threat has passed, the response may continue to smolder. In fact, the unending stress of modern life keeps millions of Americans perpetually living in just such a simmering crisis state.

ADRENAL BURNOUT

When this happens, the adrenal glands eventually become exhausted. A pair of endocrine glands atop each kidney, the adrenals secrete hormones that regulate key functions of the energy process. Glucocorticosteroid hormones control the metabolism of food into energy. Cortisol maintains the liver's role in regulating the blood sugar level. Other glucocorticosteroids regulate muscle integrity and control mineral balance.

From the medulla or interior part of the adrenals come adrenalin, noradrenalin and dopamine, catecholamine hormones that control the fight or flight response.

Together with the thyroid gland, the adrenals form the very core of the body's energy mechanism. Obviously, the fight or flight response consumes energy. But when the adrenals are continually excited by unresolved emotional stress, they may become fatigued. Stress hormones remain in the blood stream, as the body continues to function in a crisis mode, its energy resources draining away.

When reduced to basics, chronic tiredness translates into perennially tired muscles. I'm not only talking about physical energy which is the ability to perform physical work. The brain is also powered by the same energy. Thus elevating your physical energy may also improve your memory, concentration, ability to make decisions and other mental functions.

Unfortunately, our twentieth century culture is geared to nonexertion and to turning us into a nation of couch potatoes. Anyone who totally accepts the modern lifestyle, and surrenders his or her vitality to automobiles and machines, is fairly guaranteed to lose all strength and stamina and to become chronically fatigued.

OUR PRIMATE HERITAGE

The explanation became clearer in 1988 when both British and American anthropologists announced that some 99 percent of man's genes were identical to those of a chimpanzee and other higher primates. Until eight million years ago, both man and other higher primates shared the same common ancestors.

Most of our genes evolved during 60 million years of life as arboreal primates. Over the millenia, our tails and some of our hair have disappeared and we have flatter faces. But few anthropologists believe that our organs and other physiology have changed significantly since paleolithic times.

Excluding our brains, we have inherited the physiology of a plant-eating higher primate. The genes in each of our cells evolved from meeting the needs of a physically-active lifestyle spent gathering fruits and other plant foods in a primeval forest.

Most of us forget that we still consist of cells that flourish on an active lifestyle and that draw most of their energy from the same plant-based foods on which our ancestors thrived. Even a century ago, most people were still following fairly simple lifestyles based on physical exertion and homegrown foods. But now, suddenly, in just a few decades, we have been thrown into a hi-tech, urban lifestyle that is completely alien to our primate bodies.

THE STRESSED-OUT SOCIETY

Most of us fail to recognize what is happening because it occurs so gradually. But to stay abreast of foreign competition, American corporations have become obsessed with forging humans into robot-like mechanisms for industrial production. Many jobs have become so dehumanizing and repetitive that millions call in sick, unable to face another stressful day.

Other millions are unable to keep up with new equipment and the constantly stepped-up pace. Every year, stress forces millions to retire from high pressure jobs at age 55.

At home, Americans must face a fresh set of problems. Many are overwhelmed by bills, unexpected repair costs and medical expenses, and the need to take out more loans to cover college costs and the burden of supporting aging parents.

When we must struggle continually with conflicts like these our human minds may find solutions but all too often, our primate bodies are depleted of energy and chronically fatigued.

Surveys show that thousands of baby boomers have become so accustomed to stress that many feel incomplete without it. Actually, they have become so addicted to adrenalin that they actively seek out stressful situations. By always having a new crisis to cope with, they can depend on experiencing a fresh adrenal high and its accompanying energy flush. As you can probably guess, though, a few months of these yo-yo effects seriously abuse and overtax the adrenals, often leading to clinical depression or disease.

In our culture, the opposite of an adrenalin junkie is a person who holds only positive, health-enhancing beliefs. By holding only optimistic expectations for the future, such a person is motivated to eat healthful low-fat foods, to exercise daily and to perceive the world as a friendly, nonthreatening place. Rarely, if ever, does a physically active person like this experience chronic weariness. Surveys show that, almost invariably, chronic tiredness strikes only sedentary people with a pessimistic outlook and poor health habits.

Thus far, this chapter has covered a wide array of topics, from belief systems to lifestyle problems. Together, they create a complex interplay of factors that affect our minds, moods and energy. Even psychologists are not quite sure how it all works out in the mind. But one thing seems certain: eventually, the typical stressed-out American experiences a mild level of depression and anxiety.

DEFUSING MILD DEPRESSION AND ANXIETY

I'm not talking about clinical depression, a major depressive disorder which requires medical treatment. Nor do I mean chronic low-grade depression. Either of these conditions, along with chronic anxiety, should have already been detected by your doctor during your medical checkup (see Chapter 2).

In contrast to these more serious disorders is mild depression, or mild anxiety, neither of which is normally serious enough to require antidepressants or psychiatric counseling. Many people with mild depression do not feel sad and the only symptoms are chronic fatigue and poor self-esteem. Most people with mild depression are not even aware that they are depressed. Yet almost everyone with chronic tiredness has some degree of mild depression or anxiety. And mild as these dysfunctions seem, they can have a profound effect on our ability to think and act.

For instance, their depressed outlook has led millions of people with chronic tiredness to lose their ability to make choices or decisions, or to act or exert themselves physically. They also have lost much of their interest in activities they previously enjoyed. No longer do they have any goals or expectations for the future. And they have entirely lost their motivation.

How can a person who is unwilling to act or to exert

themselves ever overcome chronic fatigue? How can a person without expectations or goals ever become sufficiently motivated to adopt the Fatigue Fighter techniques in this book?

These are valid concerns.

Nevertheless, by allowing you to intervene at every level in the energy process—from replacing destructive beliefs to adopting a high-energy diet—the Fatigue Fighter techniques enable you to practice a powerful form of behavioral medicine. From restoring your motivation and your ability to act and move to relaxing the adrenals and revitalizing weak muscles, the 18 Fatigue Fighters rebuild your ability to tap into your energy resources at every level of the bodymind.

Once the desire to act and move exists in the mind, the rest is up to the digestive and muscular systems.

THE KREBS CYCLE

For literally millions of years, our primate ancestors lived by gathering fruits, vegetables, legumes and whole grains for food. In view of this evolutionary background, it is hardly surprising that carbohydrates from plant foods continue to remain the body's preferred energy source.

The series of biochemical reactions through which our bodies metabolize carbohydrates into energy to fuel the muscles is known to scientists as the Krebs Cycle.

After being digested, the starches and sugars in plant foods are broken down into glucose, a form of sugar. As this glucose enters the bloodstream, the pancreas normalizes the blood sugar level by releasing insulin. Insulin lowers the blood sugar level by converting surplus glucose into glycogen for storage in muscles, cells and liver.

51

Excluding diabetics, this process is active in virtually every living person. Thus, regardless of how chronically tired we are, our energy resources are usually still intact.

So what prevents us from tapping into this energy? Not surprisingly, perhaps, it's our old friends, the adrenal glands. The adrenals are responsible for releasing and mobilizing our stored-up glycogen energy reserves. But in many people with chronic tiredness, the adrenals have been so fatigued by constant stress that they are unable to secrete sufficient hormones to do the job.

BEATING THE LOW BLOOD SUGAR BLUES

When we draw on glucose in the bloodstream for energy, our blood sugar level falls. In a healthy person, this is a signal for the adrenals to secrete adrenalin and other hormones. These hormones then signal the liver and muscle cells to convert some of their stored-up glycogen back into glucose and release it into the bloodstream. In this way, a falling blood sugar level is restored to normal.

But when the adrenals are fatigued by stress, they are unable to release the required hormones and our muscles are starved for energy. Worsening the situation is the fact that the adrenals also secrete key hormones essential to the metabolism of carbohydrates, fats, and proteins, and for the integrity of muscles.

Efficient carbohydrate metabolism is essential because carbohydrates from plants are the principal source of fuel for the muscles. The carbohydrates we're talking about are those found in fresh fruits, vegetables, whole grains, and legumes, and in nuts and seeds—in other words, in whole, unprocessed plant foods exactly as they exist in nature.

COMPLEX CARBOHYDRATES TO THE RESCUE

These foods are known as complex carbohydrates because each consists of living cells. Each cell is enclosed by a cellulose wall. Since cellulose breaks down slowly in the human digestive tract, the starches and sugars in complex carbohydrates are released at a slow but steady rate. The pancreas is easily able to release sufficient insulin to normalize the blood sugar level. And a meal of complex carbohydrates liberates sufficient energy to fuel the muscles for two to three hours of vigorous exercise.

But complex carbohydrates presented problems to the modern food industry. Whole grains and other complex carbohydrates quickly spoil if not refrigerated. To extend their shelf life, and thus increase profits, the food industry began to refine sugar, wheat and rice. The refining process strips these foods of their cellulose and of their vitamin and mineral content. What is left consists of refined or simple carbohydrates.

Consisting of little more than empty calories, and almost completely devoid of any fiber or natural nutrients, these foods are the principal type of carbohydrates eaten by Americans today. Except for white rice, which isn't quite as depleted, no other refined carbohydrate can be recommended as a desirable energy source.

THE CHEMISTRY OF MUSCLE FUELS

When you begin to walk, or to perform any other rhythmic exercise, for the first 20 minutes your muscles draw exclusively on energy from carbohydrate foods. Then, slowly but gradually, your muscles tap into fat in the bloodstream for energy.

After exercising for an hour, for instance, 15 percent of your calories are likely to be supplied by fat compared to 85 percent from carbohydrates. The longer the duration of your walk or workout, the more calories you consume from fat and the fewer from carbohydrates. After two hours, for instance, you might typically be drawing 25 percent of calories from fat and only 75 percent from carbohydrates. The reason is that your glycogen reserves are being used up and you must draw increasingly on fat for energy.

Fat, then, is the body's second choice muscle fuel. And the average American certainly has plenty to draw on. In the ideal diet, not more than 15 to 20 percent of calories should be from fat while 65 to 70 percent should be from complex carbohydrates. But in the standard American diet, a whopping 39 percent of calories are derived from fat while a mere 42 percent are from carbohydrates. And unfortunately, most of those carbohydrates are refined. The bulk of the American diet consists of fat, white flour and sugar plus about three times as much protein as the body needs. (Since protein cannot be stored in the body, it has little value as a muscle fuel.)

The prevailing opinion of most sports nutritionists today is that a diet this high in fat and this low in carbohydrates cannot possibly maintain an optimal level of glycogen for powering muscles. Yet the majority of Americans continue to eat a diet destined to provide them with substandard energy.

PROVOCATIVE FINDINGS

A recent study by the CDC revealed that only 9 percent of Americans eat a total of five helpings of fresh fruits and vegetables per day—the bare minimum for healthful nutrition. This implies that 91 percent of Americans get their energy from a combination of refined carbohydrates and fat. And most of that consists of candy disguised as breakfast cereals, white bread and other baked goods made from white flour, ice cream, and twice as much fat and oil as the body can comfortably tolerate.

Unlike complex carbohydrates, which break down and release their starch and sugar gradually, white flour and white sugar release their calories almost immediately. This rush of glucose overloads the ability of the pancreas to secrete insulin. Without sufficient insulin, the blood sugar level soars. Instead of being stored as glycogen, the glucose remains in the bloodstream.

Granted, there is glucose aplenty—for a brief while! But as the muscles burn up this bloodstream glucose, the blood sugar level plummets. And glycogen reserves are then insufficient to restore the blood sugar level.

Anyone who is walking or using his muscles, or even sitting down, may suddenly feel drained of energy. Most people recognize this state as a condition of low blood sugar. Others, who may experience irritability, poor concentration, headaches or mood swings along with flagging energy, often call it hypoglycemia.

Most doctors today agree that hypoglycemia is rarely a dysfunction but is merely a normal function of the energy mechanism. Even people who eat complex carbohydrates exclusively eventually run low on energy and experience hunger.

55

THE DESTRUCTIVE EFFECT OF DEVITALIZED FOODS

Low blood sugar is seldom considered a medical condition because the cure is simple. You can end it in minutes by eating or drinking a carbohydrate snack. Fastest to act is a sugar-laden drink or a glass of fruit juice or a tablespoon or so of honey or other natural sweetener. Each of these, incidentally, is a refined carbohydrate.

Millions of Americans depend on doughnuts and coffee, or a candy bar, for their next energy "fix." When you use more refined carbohydrates to overcome low blood sugar you simply create a repeat of the same low blood sugar cycle. Another Danish and more coffee is guaranteed to send the blood sugar level soaring again, only to have it plummet once more in less than an hour.

More than any other organ, the brain depends on a high blood sugar level for efficient operation. And this organ reacts swiftly to a drop in blood sugar. Ability to think or to concentrate and to make sound judgments and choices is immediately impaired. People who depend on refined carbohydrates for their energy frequently become addicted to sugar and white flour. After a few years of roller-coaster blood sugar levels, they become likely candidates for impaired immunity or for diabetes or depression.

THE THREE O'CLOCK SLUMP

Every afternoon at about three o'clock, millions of men and women find their energy flagging. Scientists call it the "postprandial dip." By midafternoon, many people feel more like napping than working. And their energy dips to its low of the day.

Here again, low blood sugar is the culprit and almost invariably, the cause turns out to be a combination of refined carbohydrates and a stimulant such as caffeine. Surveys have shown that the majority of people who experience postprandial dip typically have a sweet roll and coffee for breakfast with another doughnut and coffee at midmorning and a combination of fat, white bread and more coffee for lunch.

Fortunately, FF#11-A (Energy Booster #8: Eliminate the Postprandial Dip) should effectively end the three o'clock slump once and for all. But the extent to which it is experienced reveals our widespread dependence on stimulants.

People's addiction to both caffeine and nicotine stems from the ability of these drugs to stimulate the adrenal glands, and to get the adrenal hormones flowing to liberate energy. This works for a brief time but only at the cost of fatiguing the adrenals even more. Within 30 minutes the adrenals are drooping again and energy is sagging. Several times each day, throughout the world, at least a billion people compulsively depend on coffee, tea or cigarettes for an energy "fix."

When the adrenals are badly fatigued, a person addicted to an adrenalin "high" may need to chain smoke, or to drink a strong cup of coffee every 30 minutes, to get the adrenal hormones briefly flowing once more.

Obviously, no one who smokes, or is addicted to caffeine, can hope to become a high-energy person. Chapter 7 may help to break dependence on stimulants.

HIGH-ENERGY DUO: ATP AND COENZYME Q-10

The final link in the energy mechanism occurs when muscle cells transform glucose and fatty acids in the bloodstream into mechanical energy. For this to happen, a series of essential nutrients must be available every step of the way. That includes not only important vitamins and minerals but an adequate supply of cellular enzymes.

To permit glucose to enter the walls of body cells, for example, a complex grouping of insulin, the hormone cyclic AMP, and GTF (glucose tolerance factor) must each be present in the right amount. Any deficiency in these substances would force the body to turn for energy to fatty acids, or even to protein.

But before the biochemical liberation of energy can begin, two additional substances must also be present. The first is creatinine phosphate, or CP, which is stored in muscle cells. The other is coenzyme Q-10, or ubiquinine. Both are essential for the transformation of glucose into adenosine triphosphate, or ATP, the actual fuel which powers the muscles.

Since barely three ounces of ATP can exist in the body at any one time—enough to sustain a runner for a mere six or seven seconds— it must be constantly resynthesized. For this to occur, an adequate supply of coenzyme Q-10 is essential.

Coenzyme Q-10 is found in every cell of a healthy person. But in older people, or in those with heart disease, a nutritional deficiency or, perhaps a genetic defect, the body's supply of coenzyme Q-10 could be impaired. Cardiologists are just beginning to recognize that up to 75 percent of all people with heart disease may have a deficiency of coenzyme Q-10. Levels may also decrease in the body with age, leading to lethargy and fatigue in older people.

It is no exaggeration to say that an adequate supply of coenzyme Q-10 is another vital step in the body's energy mechanism. Coenzyme Q-10 is found in meat, and in fish such as mackerel and sardines, and in cereals, bran, soybeans, nuts and dark green vegetables. Some reports claim that fatigued older people, whose diets did not include these foods, have been helped by oral supplements of coenzyme Q-10.

THE MAGIC OF OXYGEN

A generous supply of oxygen is the final prerequisite in the energy process. Without adequate oxygen, brought in by the heart and lungs, ATP production falls off by as much as 85 percent. Instead of being transformed into ATP and burned for energy, glucose is changed into lactic acid and its energy is lost.

A very adequate supply of oxygen is therefore necessary before we can tap into the energy in glucose and fatty acids. Aerobic exercise requires a constant supply of oxygen. In fact, the entire focus of aerobic exercise is to increase the body's oxygen uptake. Chapter 6 demonstrates how, once aerobic fitness is achieved, you can walk or jog or bicycle or work for hours without becoming tired.

Above all else, oxygen is the key to mobilizing more energy. And Chapter 6 clearly shows how you can dramatically increase your oxygen uptake by increasing the efficiency of your cardiovascular system.

In sharp contrast, muscles deprived of oxygen swiftly become fatigued. Smoking is a guaranteed way to deprive our cells of oxygen. Almost as effective is unresolved emotional stress, which keeps the fight or flight response turned on, thus restricting breathing and constantly consuming oxygen to keep the muscles tensed.

Building up motivation, exercising, eating a high-energy diet, and overcoming stress, are all action steps that work together to end chronic tiredness. Relatively few people are fortunate enough to discover a single magic bullet, just one step, that alone will restore their energy. For those who do, however, that magic bullet is usually exercise. Regular aerobic exercise is the one step that, alone, can overcome chronic tiredness for good.

By studying Chapter 6, and beginning a graduated aerobic exercise program, a formerly fatigued person can become charged with energy in just a few weeks.

To rebuild your energy, you must first expend energy. By exercising the cardiovascular system and becoming fit, you can dramatically increase the oxygen supply to your muscle cells. Tasks that may seem exhausting now may soon become easy. And in a few weeks, chronic tiredness can become just a memory.

AN ACTION-STEP THAT LIFTS YOUR SPIRITS

Furthermore, by exercising aerobically each day for 30 minutes or more, most people experience a wonderful euphoria that lasts the rest of the day. Known as "runner's high," it occurs as rhythmic exercise releases clouds of endorphins in the brain. These stimulating neurotransmitters bind with pain receptors in the brain, virtually blocking out any feeling of pain. As a result, we feel only pleasure. And we continue to experience elation, usually until we fall asleep.

Incidentally, any rhythmic exercise maintained for 30 minutes or longer should produce "runner's high." Brisk walking, jogging, bicycling, swimming, cross-country skiing, even canoe paddling, should all result in uplifted spirits. The effect is so predictable that a number of psychiatrists have found exercise to be more effective in beating depression than either drugs or counseling.

YOUR ENERGY: USE IT OR LOSE IT

Once your energy has been restored, you must keep on expending it through regular exercise. At any time you stop exercising for more than a few days, a feeling of lassitude spreads throughout the bodymind and you begin to lose the ability to tap into your energy resources.

We must never forget that our primate bodies can flourish and remain healthy only when we lead the vigorous, active lifestyle for which our genes evolved. As soon as we stop exercising regularly, and exerting our muscles, our entire energy mechanism becomes sluggish. This lassitude reaches into every area of the bodymind. Our good intentions are overwhelmed by complacency. In no time at all, we're back on the couch watching TV. And once again, we have lost the ability to tap into our energy resources.

Still another energy maxim states: "The body supplies us with all the energy for our needs." All too often, the reason we have no energy is because our lifestyle is so sedentary that it places no demands for energy.

Let's say, for example, that your muscles are all charged up with glycogen and ATP and coenzyme Q-10. Your mus-

61

cles and joints are in perfect shape. You are assured that you could easily walk a brisk ten miles without any physical problems or discomfort whatever. The weather is mild, sunny and calm.

Outside is a smoothly-paved hiking trail that loops past beautiful woods and lakes and over hill and dale for ten full miles. There is absolutely no chance of your experiencing tiredness, heat, cold, thirst, hunger or any kind of inconvenience. It's all perfectly safe, free of dogs, insects, people or any other possible drawback or danger. And you can't get lost.

Remember, your muscles have more than enough energy for this hike. But you must walk it alone.

Given a full day off from work, which one of the following three activities would you prefer:

1. Walk the ten mile hiking trail.
2. Spend your time strolling around a shopping mall.
3. Stay indoors and watch TV.

If your answer is #2 or #3, and you're frequently tired and low on energy, you may very well have discovered the reason for your weariness.

Generally, the body supplies us with all the energy we demand. But if our lifestyle is built around TV-viewing, or visiting shopping malls, or watching spectator sports, it creates little or no demand for energy. And that's exactly what we get: little or no energy!

To become a high energy person means doing some rethinking, from rethinking what a plate of healthy food looks like to rethinking our attitudes about exercise and about TV-watching or shopping at the mall. Chapter 12 is filled with guidelines for creating a high-energy lifestyle in which fatigue is unknown.

62

IS SLEEP STARVATION ROBBING YOU OF VIGOR?

Sleep starvation may not directly impair the energy mechanism. But it's another energy drain that we could all do without.

In today's helter-skelter world, millions who moonlight and work overtime find that sleep is the most readily expendable way to get more time. Untold numbers of Americans sleep only four to six hours each night and many build up a severe sleep deficit. Sleep-starved people frequently feel drowsy during the day and both their physical and mental performance suffer.

A recent study at Henry Ford Hospital's Sleep Disorder and Research Center, Detroit, found that a person's alertness could be increased 25 percent by adding an hour of extra sleep each night.

A good indicator is that if you need an alarm to wake up, you are not getting enough sleep. Chapter 10 tells how to guarantee yourself adequate sleep and it also describes how to wake up each morning full of pep and rarin' to go.

HOW GENDER AND AGE AFFECT CHRONIC FATIGUE

Women appear to experience chronic fatigue twice as often as men, leading some doctors to speculate that women may be more willing than men to discuss it.

Age seems to have little relationship to chronic weariness. Today, many people of 75 have double the energy of other people who are half their age. However, in an older person with chronic tiredness, it may take somewhat longer to restore energy. One reason is that, the older a person is, the longer he or she may have abused the adrenals and bodymind.

Nonetheless, given the willingness to act, you can rebuild your energy at any age.

CHAPTER FIVE

Boost Your Motivation with Behavioral Medicine

H ow many psychologists does it take to change a light bulb?

Only one. But the bulb must be willing to change.

This quip from the '60s reminds us that to restore our energy we must be willing to relinquish the "benefits" of chronic tiredness. Millions of Americans have become emotionally dependent on, or attached to, chronic fatigue. They have found that it can save them from any kind of physical exertion or from having to do volunteer work or even housework.

One survey found that a person who talks a lot about

chronic fatigue, visits a series of doctors (none of whom can find anything wrong), and tries one passive remedy after another, may have developed an emotional investment in the condition.

For those who are genuinely willing to let go of chronic tiredness, but whose motivation may seem weak, this chapter introduces us to behavioral medicine.

Unlike cognitive positivism, which changes the way we feel by changing the way we believe and think, behavioral medicine changes the way we feel by changing the way we act.

Some people find it easy to psych themselves up to act and begin a self-help program. But behavioral medicine warns the majority of us not to count on an avalanche of motivation anytime soon.

ACTION OVERCOMES FATIGUE

According to the behavioral school of psychology, action must precede motivation. Only after you have acted by adopting two or three of the Fatigue Fighter techniques will you get the motivation to adopt the rest.

Before being given the motivation to act, you must act first. This is like having to exert yourself to prime your energy mechanism before it will begin restoring your energy reserves.

The validity of the 18 Fatigue Fighter techniques has never been questioned. But all are active therapies. And some doctors and writers have questioned whether Americans have the motivation to accept the lifestyle changes which are a built-in part of these self-help techniques. This conclusion is based on the assumption that the average American is a weak-willed, self-indulgent person who wavers easily, yields to every temptation and would rather watch TV or a ball game than go for a hike.

WE ALREADY HAVE MORE MOTIVATION THAN WE THINK

While there's undoubtedly some truth here, I don't buy into this stereotyped image.

The reason is that, in recent years, over 30 million Americans have quit smoking, an accomplishment several times more difficult than adopting all of the Fatigue Fighter techniques put together.

Furthermore, studies are demonstrating that our power to change is far greater than most of us think. Leading behavioral psychologists are pointing out that the only thing that keeps us complacent is our desire to remain in the "comfort zone."

In response to the stress of growing up, each of us tends to create a comfortable lifestyle built around eating sweet and fatty foods, watching TV and avoiding most forms of physical exertion. Put together, these indulgences form our "comfort zone." As we grow up, we tend to regard it as "the good life."

For example, eating is a nurturing and comforting social act. Most of us continue to eat the same foods that we grew up with, a learned behavior that becomes a deeply ingrained part of our culture.

When we reach adulthood, eating a diet high in sugar, fat

67

and protein continues to be comforting because it reinforces memories of when we were fed these same foods to comfort us as youngsters.

As we grow older, we continue to rely on these same rich, low-energy foods to comfort us and to tranquilize us against the stress of daily living. By the time we reach our 20s, we so crave being in the comfort zone that the majority of us assume we are locked into these habits for life.

FEEDBACK OPENS THE COMFORT-ZONE BARRIER

Yet the comfort zone scenario overlooks a key factor in behavioral psychology. Time and again, studies have clearly demonstrated that most people are willing to change their diet and lifestyle—as long as they begin to have more energy in just a few days.

To boost our motivation, we need almost immediate feedback.

Positive feedback, in the shape of increased energy, is exactly what you are likely to experience when you adopt the Fatigue Fighter techniques. Observations show that almost everyone who has adopted these natural therapies has experienced a steady increase in reserves of new energy. As chronic tiredness gradually fades, virtually everyone feels better than they have in years.

Kent Jones, a Denver bank loan officer, was addicted to ice cream and pastries, but he would feel energetic for only an hour after eating these refined carbohydrate foods. From then on, he would go into an energy tailspin that, for much of the day, left him totally drained and unable to concentrate or make sound decisions. Kent was warned that unless he could stabilize his energy, his employers might have to let him go.

In desperation, Kent turned to FF#10 ("Replace These Counterfeit Foods with Energy-Filled Complex Carbohydrates"). Although it meant a wrenching change, he let go of all ice cream, sugar, cookies and white bread and replaced them with high energy complex carbohydrates like oatmeal with fresh fruit, and combinations of beans with potatoes, sweet potatoes, millet and rice.

"I couldn't believe the difference," Kent told us. "In just four days, my energy level stabilized and my low blood sugar disappeared. I was so elated that I immediately started a walking exercise program. And in just ten more days my energy level had doubled again."

SUCCESS IS THE BEST MOTIVATOR

Success is the best of all possible motivators. As Kent discovered, in just a short time, the Fatigue Fighter techniques may so boost energy that any sacrifice seems insignificant by comparison.

All this adds up to a cogent argument against the almost universal assumption that most Americans are unwilling or unable to adopt and stay with the Fatigue Fighter techniques. Instead, motivational studies have clearly proved that success is the best of all possible motivators. Most people are powerfully motivated by concern for their health and quality of life. And to restore their energy, the majority are clearly willing to step outside their comfort zone.

Most of us, in fact, are far hardier and more flexible and adaptable than we give ourselves credit for. Most men and women have the potential to become survivors—for example, to survive being lost for days in the wilderness rather than to give up and die. Nor are we easily intimidated by mild inconveniences or by mental or physical exertion.

Using the behavioral approach, most of us are thoroughly capable of mobilizing the commitment and perseverance we need to survive. By the same token, we can beat chronic fatigue rather than giving up and remaining perennially tired.

The following three self-help techniques each use the behavioral approach to help boost motivation. FF#1 can help you break out of motivational paralysis. FF#2 describes how to win at the energy-building game. And in FF#2-A you learn how aversion therapy can help break almost any type of energy-draining addiction.

•FATIGUE FIGHTER #1: Empowering Yourself to Overcome Motivational Paralysis

Mild depression does not invariably accompany chronic tiredness. But when it does, it may manifest as a do-nothing lethargy commonly known as motivational paralysis. This apathy can be so severe that a person with chronic fatigue may stubbornly refuse to do anything to help herself. While in this condition, a person may be unable to use the self-help techniques in this book.

People with motivational paralysis seem to have no energy, even for small routine tasks such as washing dishes, taking a shower or cleaning the refrigerator. So overpowering is their inertia that they avoid having to act or move or to make any

70

decisions. They become victims of a vicious cycle of passivity that endlessly maintains their state of chronic tiredness.

For some years, behavioral psychologists have known that motivation eludes many people with chronic fatigue. Even if a fatigued person fortifies himself with high-energy foods plus vitamins, minerals and co-enzyme Q-10, he may still not feel motivated or energetic.

The behavioral approach assumes that we can change the way we feel by the way we act. Thus action must precede motivation. To break the vicious cycle of inertia, we must act first. When we act, motivation follows. In this way, the decision to help oneself by acting is the key to overcoming chronic tiredness.

We must realize that it is only our motivation that is paralyzed. After all, we can get up at any time to go to the bathroom. We are not physically paralyzed. It's simply our motivation that is frozen. Hence by getting up and doing something, such as walking around the block, we can unlock our motivation and boost our self-esteem.

The trick, of course, is to urge a fatigued person to act in the first place. So let's assume that you have some degree of motivational paralysis. Now that you know there will be a reward, deciding to act should be much less difficult.

ACTION TAPS YOUR HIDDEN ENERGY

So choose an action. Preferably decide on something which involves some physical exertion. Remember, you have to prime the pump. To build up your energy you have to expend some energy first. Probably the best action you can choose is to take a short walk: for five minutes or around the block or just a hundred yards, whatever feels comfortable. Now focus your mind on the action. Close your eyes and visualize yourself taking the walk. Then get up and DO IT!

If you did take that walk, you now understand that it was the attempt to act that, in mere minutes, transformed your mood from feeling blue to feeling exuberant. Merely making a genuine attempt to act can cause us to smile instead of feel sad, and to stand upright instead of slouching.

If you still couldn't make the attempt to walk, or to act, then try this approach. Take a pen and pad and write down two things you must do today. Then make sure you do them.

If writing a list seems to help, consider making a list of every activity you should do today. Begin with something you've been putting off, like phoning the dentist for an appointment or paying a bill or writing a letter to someone. Then include all routine chores on your list.

Each day, go through the list and tick off each item as you do it. Next, begin to add small, readily achievable goals such as walking for five minutes.

Without a written list, fatigued people can feel overwhelmed by undone tasks and unresolved decisions. The next step is to make a list of all the larger jobs you must do. Write each task on a separate index card. Then give each a number, thus:

1 = urgent, do now
2 = priority, don't postpone
3 = do fairly soon
4 = not needed yet

Sort the cards into piles by number. Then put aside those numbered 2, 3 and 4. As your energy level rises, begin adding one or two of the number one tasks to your daily list. And as your energy increases, add some new and exciting activities, especially on weekends.

Make your initial task some simple, easy chore you have been putting off for weeks, like cleaning out a drawer or paying a bill or writing a letter you owe someone. Even though you may not exert your muscles, once you have acted, you will begin to feel better than you have in weeks.

RESTORE YOUR ABILITY TO MAKE SOUND CHOICES

Next, try making a choice or decision you have been putting off.

Let's say you bought 200 shares of a stock at $20 and it has risen in value to $50. You can't decide whether to sell now and lock in your profit or to wait and see if the price goes higher still. If you do wait, of course, the risk is that the price could fall, causing you to lose some of your gain.

To make any logical choice, one should first find out everything one can about the situation. Where stocks are concerned, no one is ever certain what the market or any individual issue will do. Hence the logical choice is to lock in half your profit by selling half your shares. Should the price drop, your losses are halved. And if the price rises, half your original shares will continue to gain in value.

To make a rational choice like this, and to act on it by calling your broker, is to break the spell that is paralyzing your motivation and keeping you frozen in lethargy and indecision. For example, you now have the power to choose to use the Fatigue Fighter methods in this book to help you overcome chronic tiredness.

Two additional therapeutic steps can help you outsmart motivational paralysis.

73

First, make restoring your energy your top priority. To do this, you cannot keep your options open. Trying to achieve several goals simultaneously can spread your energy thin. It takes a clear and undivided intention to act to overcome inertia and lethargy. So until you beat chronic tiredness, we suggest relegating other goals to second place—or forsaking them entirely.

PUT ATTRIBUTIONAL THERAPY TO WORK

Secondly, harness the power of attributional therapy. This is a powerful psychological benefit that appears automatically whenever you learn to attribute success in improving your energy and health to your own efforts and not to the passive reception of a drug or a treatment prescribed by someone else.

Studies show that as soon as you change a habit that produces a noticeable increase in energy, attributional therapy comes into play. It does so by providing new and powerful confirmation that you are in full control of your life and health, and that you yourself can do more to overcome chronic tiredness than can any drug or a treatment given you by someone else.

Another aspect of attributional therapy is the realization that if you can force yourself to exercise and you then feel wonderful, your chronic tiredness is seldom due to any physiological problem but only to your motivational paralysis.

As soon as you start to act and move, you should begin to feel so alive and energized that you will wonder why you were ever content to feel fatigued.

•FATIGUE FIGHTER #2: Harnessing Your Win-Power to Break Energy-Destroying Habits

You may not have motivational paralysis, but plain, every-day complacency can still prevent you from acting to overcome chronic tiredness. We all want to restore our energy but preferably without having to exercise, or having to eat more vegetables and grains, or having to learn to beat stress. Although most of us probably have some idea of how to combat chronic fatigue, many of us are too complacent to act. Too many of us have been couch potatoes all our lives and we're resistant and reluctant to change. However, by using what behavioral psychologists call "generalization of effect," changing a habit becomes almost as easy as switching to a new TV channel.

Our addiction to being in the "comfort zone" can make cutting out an old, familiar habit, or starting a new one, feel rather stressful. Even though a habit may be sapping our energy, every bone and muscle in our body seems to resist a change. It always seems easier, safer and more secure to stay the way we are. Even if we do make a change, there is no guarantee that we'll have more energy.

We all know the familiar excuses.

"It won't work."

"I've always been this way."

"I can't help it, that's the way I am."

"I'm too old to change."

"Not now, I haven't time. Perhaps next month."

Each of these excuses identifies a "loser" state of mind. We stay with our old familiar ways of living and eating because we continue to think in a "losing" way. Yet the moment we decide to step out of our "loser" attitude and start becoming a "winner," we immediately conquer all the barriers that are blocking our success.

75

WIN BACK YOUR ENERGY

Behavioral psychologists have found that almost any person can transform his personality from "loser" to "winner" in just a few minutes. Or, with practice, in just 60 seconds.

This discovery is based on the concept that you can transfer success in any one area of your life to any other area of your life. Here's how to put "generalization of effect" to work to help change some of the habits that may be contributing to chronic tiredness.

Begin by thinking about something at which you excel. It could be baseball, bowling, dancing, playing the harmonica or guitar, painting, creative writing, tennis, designing clothes, interior decorating, solving crossword puzzles or working out super-challenging logic puzzles. We all have something at which we excel and at which we know we're good.

Let's say, for example, that you recently spent a vacation riding a mountain bicycle downhill from some of the highest elevations in Colorado. Each day, a van took you and other bicyclists to the lofty heights of Vail Pass or Mount Evans. At these rarified heights, they turned you loose to coast back downhill for 20 or 30 miles. Very little physical effort was required. But as the days went by, and you learned to ride over rocks and tree stumps, you became increasingly confident of your ability to ride down any trail or road in Colorado. Whatever the difficulties, whether it was snow, mud or gravel on the road, you could overcome them and win.

Now, suppose you were asked to cut out coffee, the same aromatic beverage that your van driver served you before you started on your long descent down the mountain each morning. It's the same coffee that gets you going every morning, that keeps the postprandial dip at bay each afternoon and that supplies a lift after dinner.

This is the same coffee that stimulates your adrenals and keeps draining your energy and that prevents you from getting to sleep. Somehow, the "loser" aspect of your personality still prefers the temporary pleasure of several cups of coffee each day, even though you know it is sapping your energy. You find it difficult to try and break this comfortable, familiar habit.

HARNESSING WIN-POWER TO END FATIGUE

Start right now by relaxing. Visualize yourself back high in the mountains. See your bike glide forward as you soar effortlessly downhill. Feel the wind and sun on your face as you ride your bike expertly down a narrow trail. Recall the tremendous build-up of power you experienced at the realization that you could travel 20 or 30 miles through the mountains without relying on gasoline power.

Relive again all the cheerfulness, optimism, confidence, persistence and aliveness that, during the bike rides, made you a "winner." Analyze and identify this win-power state of mind. Hold on to that feeling.

Next, slide the bike scene off your inner video screen and create a vivid picture of yourself sipping your after-dinner coffee. Recall the rich aroma and how good it tastes. Then switch immediately to another scene of yourself in bed, fitfully tossing and turning and unable to sleep. Recall how the coffee is stressing your adrenals and depriving you of needed sleep. Recall how bad it feels.

Above all, realize that but for your chronic tiredness, you

77

might have bicycled *up* those mountains as well as down. Make a silent commitment that, more than anything else, you want to stop drinking coffee. Then release all that win-power you just mobilized in the biking scenes. Transfer it to your commitment to cut out coffee now.

Feel the irresistible win-power surge within you as you commit yourself to giving top priority in your life to ending the coffee habit. Eliminating coffee is now the most important thing in your life. You have a passionate, crusading zeal to kick the coffee habit once and for all.

You know that nothing can stand in the way of your success. You have transferred the same win-power you developed in bicycling to another area of your life—breaking the caffeine habit. Don't be surprised if you hurry to the kitchen and tip your remaining coffee into the garbage.

For at least the next week or two, your newfound zeal must be regularly reinforced. Each time you feel the urge to drink coffee, you must repeat this win-power imagery. Each time it will become easier and each time your win-power will become stronger and more persistent.

PRACTICE BEHAVIORAL MEDICINE YOURSELF

Each time you use this win-power technique you are practicing behavioral medicine. By breaking a destructive habit and replacing it with an energy-building habit, you are training and exercising your mind in a similar way to that in which we train and exercise our bodies. As the mind builds new neural pathways, and new ways of believing and thinking, you will suddenly find yourself free of the coffee habit just as you once suddenly discovered you could swim or ride a bicycle.

78

In Chapter 4 you learned that age is no barrier to overcoming chronic tiredness. Nor is age a barrier to using win-power. Once you create the win-power mind state, you can adopt any of our Fatigue Fighters at any age. It's never too late to change until you give up.

After practicing the win-power visualization several times, you'll find you can psych yourself up into a winning mindstate in barely one minute. The more frequently you enter the win-power mind state, the easier it becomes to remain at this exuberant level permanently.

•FATIGUE FIGHTER #2-A: Using Aversion Therapy to Stop Energy-Depleting Addictions

Many energy-depleting habits are hard to beat because people are addicted to them. Based on studies in behavioral motivation at Purdue and Indiana State Universities, the simple action steps described below can help you break both physical and psychological addiction to things you may crave, such as caffeine, alcohol, cigarettes, sugar, refined carbohydrates, overeating, an adrenal "high" or an aversion to exercise. Each of these habits is counter-productive and suppresses your energy.

But first, let's learn the STOP! technique. This step may sound simplistic. But don't let that obscure its power.

To get started, wear a loose-fitting rubber band around your left wrist (or your right wrist if you're left-handed). Whenever you are about to do something which you recognize as harmful or addictive, use one hand to snap the rubber band. If you don't have a band, pinch your wrist with the other hand. Then call out "Stop!" Say it aloud if you're alone or silently if others are present. Next, while you relax, take six, slow, deep breaths. Each time you exhale, repeat the word "Stop!"

This strategy—designed to change the way we feel by the way we behave—gives us time to stop and recognize our mistake. If we feel at all uncomfortable or guilty, that's a strong indication that we are about to indulge in an energy-robbing addiction.

STOPPING AN ADDICTION IN ITS TRACKS

Let's say that you are addicted to eating three large sugary doughnuts together with two cups of strong coffee for lunch each day. You recognize that this refined carbohydrate-stimulant combination is the probable cause of the letdown you experience late each afternoon. Yet your addiction is so powerful that you cannot pass the doughnut shop door without going in.

At lunch time next day, walk up as usual to the doughnut shop door. Then call out "Stop!" Snap your rubber band or pinch your wrist. Go no further. Stand still and take six deep, slow breaths. During each exhalation, tell yourself "Stop!" With each lungful of air, your willpower will grow. At the sixth exhalation, turn around and walk back up the street about 35 yards.

Then walk back to the doughnut shop, snap the band, call out "Stop!" and repeat the entire routine.

Repeat it ten times in all.

At this point, go into a salad bar and have a healthful lunch. Or bring a wholesome brown bag repast.

You may have to repeat this exercise during three or four more lunch periods. But as this powerful technique builds new neural pathways in your brain, your former "comfort zone" addiction will swiftly fade away.

USING AVERSION THERAPY TO GET BACK ON TRACK

What if, a week or a month later, you weaken and go back into the same, or another, doughnut shop. Or perhaps you may light up a cigarette, take an alcoholic drink or shun your regular exercise period.

If this happens, use aversion therapy to get back on track. One weak moment isn't going to destroy all the progress you have made.

Snap your rubber band. Call out "Stop!" Take six slow, deep breaths. And remember the principle of behavioral medicine: you can change the way you feel by the way you act. So act and throw away whatever it is that you addictively crave.

Realize that you may have become temporarily discouraged because you felt tired, tense, lonely or hungry. Every day, millions of Americans go on an eating or smoking or alcohol binge in response to stress or a negative mood. As a result, almost all suffer from some degree of chronic tiredness.

People go on binges when they fall into the trap of distorted thinking. They believe that once they fall off the wagon, even for a few minutes, they are doomed to stay there. It seems easier to keep on indulging than to climb back aboard.

Never fall into this trap. One doughnut or one cigarette

or one beer isn't going to stop you from a lifetime of new energy-building habits.

Whenever you feel like slipping back into an addiction, bolster your motivation by reading through this action-step again.

Some motivational programs allow you to deliberately "cheat" on one day each week. But most behavioral psychologists agree that cheating merely creates guilt, an unnecessary emotion that undermines your win-power spirit.

If you find yourself in a social situation where you prefer not to offend your hostess, you may occasionally be forced to "cheat." But compensate immediately by cutting back on fat or sugar (or whatever) even more for the next several days.

And do get back on track right away.

KEEP A DIARY

For anyone who enters totally into the Fatigue Fighter program, positive feedback should appear within seven to ten days. A daily written record is the best way to keep track of your progress. Keep a record of your mood and stress level and the action steps you are following. Note your progress in exercise, upgrading diet and nutrition, and cutting back on stimulants and improving sleep. Keep a record of the distance you walk each day and of your weight and resting pulse rate and of how much more energy you have with each passing day.

Each day, you'll be encouraged by seeing your progress on paper. And you'll have a written reminder of the benefits of overcoming chronic tiredness naturally.

A diary can also help you examine any negative feelings

that might come up. Occasionally, people say they feel deprived or restricted when they give up favorite foods. But most people who switch to a high-energy diet report it was never necessary to sacrifice the enjoyment of taste. They simply discovered new and exciting taste experiences from less harmful foods.

Others have told us that after beginning a daily walk they became so addicted to the exhilarating "high" that it produced that they deliberately sought out additional exercise that made them feel even better.

Instead of being addicted to your comfort zone, you can develop an addiction to the even greater comfort of possessing more energy.

CHAPTER SIX

Don't Take Fatigue Lying Down

While researching this book, I was amazed at the number of people I met who believed it was possible to be filled with energy without ever having to exercise or do anything strenuous.

It's true that some of the energy from the food you eat goes to fuel the brain and nervous system. But the majority is transformed from chemical energy into the mechanical energy that actually moves your muscles. Unless you move your body and exercise your muscles, your energy mechanism is unable to function efficiently or to produce more energy from food.

Almost any of us can create our own chronic fatigue at will simply by moving the muscles as little as possible. Spend your days on a couch watching TV, and lassitude and lethargy are virtually guaranteed.

Studies on the rigors of space flight, in which opportunities for exercise are extremely limited, have shown that sedentary living can wear out the mind and body much faster than a physically active lifestyle. A few days of physical inactivity lowers the basal metabolism, replaces muscle mass with body fat, increases loss of bone density and leads to a significant reduction in oxygen supply to body cells.

One study at Duke University Medical Center recently found that failing to exercise and to stay physically fit increased risk of heart disease and stroke to the same extent as smoking a pack of cigarettes per day.

Another study, based on a survey of 6,928 California residents by the Human Population Lab of the California Department of Health Services, found a strong relationship between symptoms of depression and lack of exercise. The study also revealed that depression symptoms quickly disappear when exercise is begun.

Depression and anxiety frequently occur in association with chronic tiredness.

PROOF THAT EXERCISE DESTROYS CHRONIC TIREDNESS

Scores of well documented studies have demonstrated that regular exercise is the one best solution for both depression and anxiety as well as for chronic tiredness. Several years ago, for instance, Dr. Harold W. Kohl of the Institute for Aerobics Research in Dallas gave treadmill walking tests to

400 out-of-shape men and women aged 30 to 65. All had reported some degree of chronic tiredness. The same tests were then repeated 30 months later. Out of 116 participants who had walked briskly several times each week during the interim, all reported reducing their levels of fatigue. Further tests showed that many of these same exercisers had lost weight, strengthened their hearts and lungs, boosted their self-esteem, and had significantly increased their stamina and endurance. The study clearly demonstrated that building and maintaining fitness by walking at a brisk pace can almost totally eliminate chronic tiredness.

Another recent study authored by William Morgan, a psychologist at the University of Wisconsin, concluded that the best antidote for anxiety is at least 20 minutes of sustained exercise, such as brisk walking, at least three times each week. Several other researchers have discovered that five 40 to 60 minutes walks or aerobic workouts per week can end mild depression sooner and more effectively than any drug or counseling treatment.

THE AMAZING HEALTH BENEFITS OF EXERCISE

Regular aerobic exercise, such as brisk walking, not only restores energy but helps to prevent heart disease, cancer, stroke, hypertension, osteoporosis and diabetes. It builds up the lean muscle mass, raising our basal metabolism and helping us to lose surplus weight. Exercise also buoys the emotions and energizes every function of both body and mind. It works like a tranquilizer to help us relax and sleep. And above all, aerobic exercise relaxes the adrenal glands and restores adrenal hormone balance; it normalizes the blood sugar level; and it improves cardiovascular and pulmonary efficiency so that the heart is able to pump more oxygen to every cell in the body with fewer beats.

In the process, exercise improves our posture, postpones aging and gives us a more youthful appearance. Studies citing these and other benefits from rhythmic exercise number in the hundreds.

Among the largest and most recent is an eight-year study of 13,000 healthy men and women by the Institute for Aerobics Research in Dallas. The study divided the participants into five groups, ranging from the most fit to the least fit. Among men, those in the least fit group died eight times more often from heart disease and four times more often from cancer than those in the most fit group. Among women, those in the least fit group died nine times more often from heart disease and 16 times more often from cancer than those who were most fit.

Another large, well-controlled study, done on some 17,000 Harvard alumni by Ralph Paffenbarger, Ph.D., concluded that men who expended 2,000 to 3,500 calories per week on exercise, such as brisk walking, reduced their risk of dying in any one year by 28 to 40 percent.

FAREWELL TO FATIGUE

Today's aerobic fitness boom is primarily about having more energy. Experience shows that men and women who take up an aerobic exercise, such as walking briskly for 30 to 45 minutes four to five times each week, generally see their chronic tiredness disappear altogether in four to six weeks. By the seventh or eighth week, they usually feel so recharged with energy that tiredness or fatigue has become just a memory.

Despite the incredible health benefits of regular exercise, a recent CDC survey found that fewer than eight percent of adult Americans exercise sufficiently to benefit their health.

Simultaneously, the CDC and other health advisory agencies pointed out that a large body of evidence exists to prove that people who fail to exercise experience not only chronic tiredness but a gradual and inexorable decline in all mind-body functions, especially in energy production. Physical and mental abilities deteriorate and rapid aging occurs. Meanwhile, scores of large population studies—each authored by a prominent scientist—have all concluded that an inactive lifestyle dramatically increases risk of every chronic disease as well as depression, anxiety and chronic fatigue.

The explanation is, of course, that our primate bodies evolved for a lifestyle of almost continuous physical activity. Instead, modern life has robbed us of our birthright by replacing almost every opportunity to exercise or exert ourselves with a power-driven machine or appliance. Our entire culture encourages us to eat more and more foods low in energy and to exercise less and less. By their early teen years, a high proportion of American youngsters have become confirmed couch potatoes. They spend their lives on the sofa, or in the car, and they abhor the outdoors. Many have mild chronic tiredness by age 15.

To win back your energy you must do the exact opposite. Regular exercise is the one action-step that can fully restore your energy. Each of the 18 Fatigue Fighter steps in this book is designed to help build up and support your energy mechanism. But in each case, the goal is to get you moving and exercising once more.

AEROBIC EXERCISE RESTORES ENERGY BEST

Several times so far I've mentioned the benefits of aerobic exercise. Aerobic exercise differs from anaerobic exercise in that its main focus is to increase oxygen uptake by the heart and lungs. Oxygen is key to mobilizing and storing more energy. Without an abundance of oxygen in the bloodstream, glucose cannot be transformed into ATP to power the body's slow-twitch muscles.

Aerobic exercise implies a continuous, rhythmic movement that uses the body's large muscle groups for a prolonged period at a speed which raises the rate of both pulse and breathing. Aerobic exercise uses the body's slow-twitch muscles, which are less powerful but can work for long periods without rest. Thus aerobic exercise includes such continuous, rhythmic endurance activities as walking, jogging, bicycling, swimming, cross-country skiing, rope-skipping or active dancing. Most stop-and-go recreations such as golf, softball, downhill skiing or doubles tennis fail to provide much aerobic benefit.

By contrast, anaerobic exercises such as weight lifting or pole vaulting employ the body's fast-twitch muscles for short bursts of energy without requiring very much oxygen. Since the fast-twitch muscles fatigue easily, anaerobic exercises fail to build up the heart and lungs or to benefit the energy mechanism.

ENRICH YOUR ENERGY WITH WALKING

Since a few weeks of sedentary living swiftly deprives the muscles of oxygen, it is aerobic exercise that we need to

89

overcome chronic tiredness. And of the various choices of rhythmic exercise, brisk walking is the one most readily available. Walking requires only a comfortable pair of shoes and most people can find somewhere close to home where walking is safe and pleasant.

If not, you might consider driving to a nearby enclosed shopping mall and walking there. Alternatively, you can swim, ride a real or stationary bicycle, skip rope or join an aerobics exercise class. However, walking on your own allows you to set your own pace and distance and to start and stop whenever you like.

If you choose walking as your aerobic exercise, we recommend purchasing a comfortable, sturdy pair of athletic fitness walking shoes from a store that specializes in sports footwear. Jogging shoes, or cross-training shoes, may serve to get started. But you'll enjoy walking much more if you wear a pair of well-cushioned shoes designed and built exclusively for fitness walking.

WHEN IT'S OK TO WALK

In Chapter 2 I recommended that you obtain your doctor's permission before beginning an exercise program. If for some reason you did not, be advised that the American College of Sports Medicine claims that if you are under 45, a non-smoker, apparently healthy, not overweight, and free from any risk factors for heart disease, you should be able to start a fairly easy but gradually-increasing exercise program without further medical screening.

Like most pro-exercise organizations, the American College of Sports Medicine is anxious to remove all potential blocks that may serve to discourage anyone from beginning to exercise.

In giving the previous advice, the College assumes that you will begin to exercise at a fairly low level of intensity, without over-exerting yourself or becoming fatigued, and that any increment will be gradual. You should always feel comfortable and avoid pushing yourself too hard (at least, until you have attained a fairly high level of cardiovascular fitness).

In releasing this information, I naturally assume that you have read Chapter 2 and have carried out its advice to obtain medical clearance before acting on anything else in this book. If you have not done so, and if you have any symptoms of chronic fatigue, I strongly recommend that you make an appointment for a medical checkup right away . . . and that you do not commence to exercise or to adopt any other action-step in this book, until you have your physician's approval.

CAUTIONS AND CAVEATS

Conversely, if you are over 45, a smoker, are overweight or have diabetes, hypertension, heart disease, elevated cholesterol or any other diagnosed illness, the American College of Sports Medicine clearly advises that you will need medical clearance from your doctor before beginning to exercise. The same caution applies if you take drugs of any kind, especially beta blockers.

Another advisory concerns males over 40 and females over 50 who may have vague chest pains, an irregular pulse, shortness of breath, a sedentary lifestyle, a family history of high cholesterol or heart disease, a high cholesterol level or a high-fat diet, and who may smoke, be overweight, have diabetes, heart disease or hypertension or who may have had rheumatic fever during childhood. Anyone in this category should also get a medical checkup with a stress test before beginning to exercise.

If at any time while exercising you experience a rapid pulse or a pounding heartbeat, extreme breathlessness, or a tightness or pain in the jaw, chest, back, shoulder, throat, or down the arm, especially on the left side, you should stop immediately. The same action is advised should you experience trembling, nausea, vomiting, dizziness, or loss of muscle control, or increasing pain in muscles and joints. These symptoms may arise because you are pushing too hard. But if they persist, see a doctor without delay.

These caveats aside, the risk of not exercising may be 1,000 times greater than any risk in taking up a gradually increasing program of brisk walking. Assuming you have observed these cautions, according to medical statistics, the risk of having a heart attack while exercising is approximately one in five million for healthy middle-aged men and one in 17 million for healthy women.

For every person who dies while exercising, 100,000 others die in bed or while smoking or eating a high-fat meal.

•FATIGUE FIGHTER #3: Walk Away Chronic Fatigue

Although exercise is the most important remedy for overcoming chronic tiredness, most fatigued people feel they lack the energy to begin.

However, very few fatigued people are unable to walk at all. At the very least they can walk to the bathroom or the length of the house. Others can walk outdoors to the mailbox and back. Often this is a distance of 40 to 50 steps.

If you're serious about overcoming chronic fatigue, you must develop your ability to walk. (Although I'm talking about walking here, the same principles apply if you are using an alternative aerobic exercise such as pedaling a stationary bicycle.)

So place a chair halfway through the house, or halfway to the mailbox. Then make the walk. After 40 steps—or however far you can comfortably go—sit down. Take half a dozen deep breaths and relax. Then when you're ready, repeat the walk. If you can walk 40 steps three times in the morning, three times in the afternoon and three more times in the evening, you'll have walked more than one-tenth of a mile, all on your first day.

To allow your muscles to recover and to rebuild their strength, walk only on alternate days. So try again two days later. Chances are good that this time you can walk 50 feet on ten different occasions—or a total of 750 feet or one-seventh of a mile.

When you exert yourself by exercising, your energy mechanism responds to this challenge by restoring the energy you have just expended *plus* a generous margin to help you go farther the next time. Thus each time you walk, you should be able to add more distance. And each time the walk will become easier and less fatiguing.

So repeat your walks on alternate days, each time striving to increase your distance and the number of times you walk. Naturally, at this stage, you should never push yourself beyond the point of comfort nor to where it hurts or you become out of breath.

Yet 12 daily walks of 110 feet each adds up to one-fourth

mile. As soon as you are able, try to walk 110 feet twice without stopping. Soon you'll be walking 220 feet six to eight times a day. Twelve walks of 220 feet each totals half a mile a day.

At this point, try to combine all your separate walks into just two or three daily walks. About three weeks after you begin, you should easily be able to walk one-fourth mile at a time without having to stop or rest or feeling exhausted. As you continue to progress, and are able to walk further each time without your muscles becoming tired, aim to combine all of your walks into a single unbroken daily walk.

It doesn't take much imagination to realize that, by the fifth week or so, you should easily be able to walk one mile at a time—and without feeling tired. Using the same principle of gradually increasing exercise just described, most people with chronic tiredness can be walking a mile within a month.

WALKING A MILE WITHOUT DISCOMFORT

When you can walk a mile at a time without discomfort, begin to increase your speed in easy, gradual stages. This may cause you to experience certain feelings that every experienced walker knows and recognizes as harmless.

While you should always be alert for the warning signs described earlier in this chapter, don't be put off by a mildly uncomfortable feeling that may appear during the first 15 to 20 minutes of exercise. This occurs as the body draws down its bloodstream glucose to fuel the muscles and it lasts until the muscles and liver begin to release their stored-up glycogen 15 to 20 minutes after exercise begins. The uncomfortable feeling occurs because the body is operating exclusively on glucose in the bloodstream.

WARM UP BEFORE WALKING

To speed up glycogen liberation, some people drink coffee before exercising. This is not recommended. Instead, you can avoid the "glucose drag" by warming up first. This means beginning to walk slowly, and gradually building up to a moderate speed over a period of five minutes or so. By then, your muscles will have warmed. So stop for a couple of minutes and do a few bends and stretches to take the stiffness out of your hips, knees and ankles. By the time you begin your regular walk, your glycogen will have kicked in and you'll be feeling great.

As you progress and are able to walk farther and faster, you'll also feel more comfortable if, at the end of your walk, you gradually slow your pace for a few minutes, then repeat the same stretches. Athletes call this the "cool-down"; it helps eliminate any muscle soreness or stiffness afterwards.

After your walk, you may experience natural tiredness. But the natural fatigue that follows a brisk walk (or a long bicycle ride or a hard tennis game) is a wonderfully relaxing feeling of satisfaction and well-being. Next morning, you will wake up feeling fully refreshed and ready to do it all again.

Natural fatigue is always replaced by energy enhancement. As you continue to gradually walk farther and faster, and your energy mechanism becomes steadily more efficient, you may experience energy enhancement in as short a time as sixty minutes after your walk ends.

By continuing to gradually increase their walking pace and

distance, most people are able to achieve a surprisingly high level of fitness and stamina within a matter of weeks. When this happens, you may also want to walk four to five times a week, or daily, instead of merely on alternate days.

By the time you can walk two to three miles, most traces of chronic tiredness should have disappeared. You may then transform yourself into a high-energy person by continuing on with FF#4.

Caution: If after following the gradually-increasing exercise program just described for a period of eight weeks, your chronic fatigue has not improved, it may be due to a dysfunction that your doctor failed to detect. In this case, return to your doctor for a further checkup.

•FATIGUE FIGHTER #4: Transform Yourself into a High-Energy Person

Assuming you have completed FF#3 and can walk two to three miles at a time without feeling tired, you should already have more energy than 50 percent of the people in the U.S. This realization usually proves so encouraging that most people are ready to go on to achieve even higher energy levels.

To become a really high-energy person, you need only to begin walking aerobically. From the frontiers of medical research, an avalanche of studies have demonstrated that an amazing transformation known as "training effect" takes place in almost everyone who takes up and stays with a structured aerobic exercise program designed to raise the pulse rate into the target zone for 30 to 50 minutes on five or more occasions each week.

Training effect takes place as the energy mechanism maximizes its aerobic capacity, meaning its ability to transport oxygen to every organ and tissue in the body.

In sedentary people, the aerobic capacity begins to decline by age 20 and by their early 60s, most inactive men and women have lost 30 to 40 percent of their aerobic capacity. In smokers, the loss is greater still. Studies by the CDC and others reveal that by age 40, millions of Americans have become so unfit that a walk around the block leaves them fatigued and out of breath.

Training effect revitalizes your energy mechanism to the point where you can rapidly inhale large amounts of air to aereate the blood. At the same time, the heart muscle develops the ability to forcefully deliver large amounts of oxygen-rich blood throughout the body.

After a few weeks of regular aerobic walking, the heart is able to pump so much more blood with each beat that your resting heart rate should drop to 65 beats per minute or less. By helping the arteries to become more flexible and relaxed, walking aerobically also helps to normalize blood pressure and cholesterol levels, to lower weight, to increase intellectual capacity and to minimize the effect of stress.

FINDING YOUR HEART RATE TARGET ZONE

To get started, calculate your personal heart target zone. To do so, subtract your age from 220. Assuming you are aged 45, this works out to 220 - 45 = 175. Thus 175 is your maximum heart rate. This pulse rate, commonly called "max," should never be exceeded.

Next, multiply your max rate by .6 and again by .8. The

resulting two figures represent 60 percent and 80 percent of max respectively. (Example: 175 × .6 = 105 or 60 percent of max; and 175 × .8 = 140 or 80 percent of max.) Thus your target heart range, or zone, is 105 to 140 beats per minute.

Training effect will now occur as you walk with your pulse rate in the heart target zone. For most of us, this means walking at a somewhat brisker pace than we're used to. For walking at this pace, we strongly urge you to observe the advice given in FF#3 for warm-up and cool-down.

To check your pulse rate while walking, stop and take your wrist pulse. Use a stopwatch to count the number of beats during a ten-second period. Begin walking immediately again while you mentally multiply your pulse count by six to get the number of beats per minute. Alternatively, you can purchase a heartbeat monitor that gives a continuous reading while you walk.

Stopping to take your pulse several times during a walk is admittedly inconvenient. But you'll have to do it at first to ensure that, while walking, your pulse remains within your heart target zone. Should your pulse fall below your target zone limit, you must increase your pace until it is again at least 60 percent of max. Or, if your pulse exceeds your zone's upper limit, you must reduce your pulse by slowing your pace.

ESTIMATING YOUR PULSE BY GUT-FEELING

The American College of Sports Medicine recently recommended that, if possible, you learn to estimate your pulse rate by gut-feeling. For example, if your workout feels "somewhat hard" your pulse is probably at 60 percent or more of max. If your pace seems "hard" you are probably at 70 percent or more of max. And if maintaining your pace seems "very hard" you are probably at 80 percent of max or over. For most people, walking at max feels "extremely hard." Whatever your level of exertion, however, you should always be able to carry on a conversation or to hum a tune without having to gasp for air.

This gut-feeling scale should help you estimate your pulse rate with some accuracy without having to stop to take your pulse or having to purchase a pulse monitor.

To begin walking aerobically, we suggest starting at a comfortable pace and gradually increasing to where you are walking briskly and staying in your heart target zone for 20 minutes on three or more occasions each week. This transition may take several weeks.

Once you can stay in your target zone for 20 minutes at a time, you can gradually increase to 25 minutes, then to 30 minutes. This is the signal to gradually increase the number of weekly workouts from three to five. Meanwhile, you can continue to gradually increase the time spent in your target zone up to 50 minutes, or slightly more, per workout.

If all this sounds rather strenuous, consider multiplying your max rate by .5 and .7. Assuming you are aged 45, this results in a heart target zone of 88 to 123 beats per minute, or 50 to 70 percent of max. Or if you prefer not to bother with target zones, merely walking at a brisk pace up and down hills can significantly boost your energy level.

The one best antidote to chronic tiredness is frequent, enjoyable, rhythmic exercise. Thus exercise should always be fun, not a form of medicine. So begin gradually and increase gradually, always avoiding discomfort, strain or excess.

By the time you can stay at 70 percent of max or over for 35 minutes at a time, training effect should be well established. Your max will have risen and so will the limits of your target heart zone.

For example, instead of having to work at 75 percent of max to walk up a hill, you'll be able to easily climb that hill at only 55 percent of max. Every physical task will become easier. You will have seemingly unlimited reserves of energy and stamina. You will stay relaxed all day and enjoy natural, unbroken sleep. And you will have more energy than 90 percent of all people in America aged over 16.

•FATIGUE FIGHTER #4-A: Become a High-Energy Superstar

Once you achieve training effect and can walk aerobically, you can reach even higher energy levels by developing the stamina and endurance to walk long distances without fatigue.

Walking with emphasis on going the distance rather than on speed is becoming increasingly popular. Over 40,000 people participate each year in Boston's 20 mile Walk for Hunger, while several hundred thousand others participate in long distance walkathons like the annual Walk America and the Super Cities Walk.

Walking 15 or 20 miles isn't as difficult as it sounds. Most coaches agree that the average walker has the stamina to cover three times the distance of a normal workout. So if you normally walk three miles, you should already have the endurance to walk nine or even ten miles. Naturally, we're talking about walking at a fairly relaxed pace, not in your target zone. And you can take short rests along the way.

BUILDING THE ENERGY TO WALK 25 MILES

To develop the energy and endurance to walk 25 miles at a stretch, most coaches use a fairly standard 42 day training schedule. Here are the distances you walk each day and the weekly totals. All Mondays are rest days.

Week 1: Tuesday 2 miles; Wednesday 3; Thursday 4; Friday 3; Saturday 4; Sunday 5; total 21.

Week 2: Tuesday 4 miles; Wednesday 5; Thursday 6; Friday 7; Saturday 4; Sunday 9; total 35.

Week 3: Tuesday 5 miles; Wednesday 6; Thursday 7; Friday 8; Saturday 5; Sunday 13; total 44.

Week 4: Tuesday 6 miles; Wednesday 7; Thursday 8; Friday 9; Saturday 6; Sunday 17; total 53.

Week 5: Tuesday 7 miles; Wednesday 8; Thursday 9; Friday 10; Saturday 7; Sunday 21; total 62.

Week 6: Tuesday 8 miles; Wednesday 9; Thursday 10; Friday 11; Saturday 5; Sunday 25; total 68.

Beginning with a walk of only two miles and a weekly total of 21, mileage increases daily to a total of 25 on the final Sunday with a weekly total of 68.

If you'd like to try this training schedule, you can either walk around a one mile loop in the park or find a longer trail. An inexpensive pedometer will monitor your daily mileage.

Most walkers find that covering any distance of 15 miles or more in a day produces levels of energy, satisfaction and well-being beyond anything that the average American can ever hope to experience.

Building the energy to walk 25 miles in a day may seem a big step from merely having the energy to walk to the bathroom. But as the saying goes, "Every thousand mile journey begins with the first step."

It won't happen overnight. Yet for anyone willing to adopt the 18 action-steps in this book, being able to eventually walk 25 miles in one day seems well within the bounds of possibility.

CHAPTER SEVEN

How Stimulants Create Chronic Tiredness by Assaulting Your Body

A lcohol, caffeine and nicotine are each a direct cause of chronic fatigue. Moreover, they have all been implicated as major causes of disturbed sleep.

Both caffeine and nicotine drain our energy by stimulating release of adrenal hormones. In the process, some of the stress mechanisms of the fight or flight response are activated, causing muscles to remain tense and to continually burn glucose and glycogen. Repeated cigarettes or cups of coffee can swiftly lead to adrenal exhaustion.

Each stimulant also works by creating satisfaction as it swiftly raises the blood sugar level. Soon, your mind is racing and you feel full of energy. But the satisfaction is short-lived. Within an hour, the blood sugar level plunges and you experience an energy slump accompanied by lethargy and fatigue.

These unpleasant feelings are actually withdrawal symptoms caused by addiction to these drugs. The only solution, it seems, is another "fix": another cup of coffee, a few more puffs on a cigarette or another alcoholic drink. Or the sugar in a candy bar or soft drink may do the trick.

Since sugar also elevates the blood sugar level, people can become as addicted to it as to the stimulants themselves. Most addicts, in fact, find that if smoking is not permitted, they can get much the same energy lift from coffee or candy. Thus smokers are often steady consumers of sugar, coffee and alcohol.

Most of us begin using caffeine or nicotine to overcome the low-energy feeling that hits us an hour or so after eating refined carbohydrates. Or we may have begun to drink coffee to get going in the morning or to offset the energy dip in mid-afternoon.

THE SECRET OF BREAKING DEPENDENCE ON STIMULANTS

Once a person becomes addicted to one or more stimulants, withdrawal can be unpleasant. Nicotine is a particularly dangerous drug addiction that is as difficult to break as being hooked on heroin or cocaine.

Whichever stimulants you're addicted to, you need to recognize that withdrawal can be much easier if you learn to keep the blood sugar level within the normal range. This avoids the periodic slump that sends you seeking another fix.

You can keep your blood sugar level out of the valleys and off the peaks by ceasing to eat refined carbohydrates in any form. Chapter 8 explains in depth the process by which white sugar, white flour and other refined grains keep the blood sugar level yo-yoing up and down. And FFs#10 and 11 give explicit instructions for eliminating these unhealthful foods from the diet and replacing them with energy-rich complex carbohydrates.

We also recommend reading Chapter 5 again and particularly FFs#1, 2 and 2-A. You will find these powerful action-steps tremendously helpful in breaking dependence on stimulants and in replacing them with the health-building exercise programs described in Chapter 6.

•FATIGUE FIGHTER #5: How To Overcome Craving For Energy-Robbing Stimulants

At any time you feel the urge for another fix of coffee, cigarettes or alcohol, these simple action-steps will help you get rid of the feeling. Remain seated and relaxed throughout.

•Step 1.

Sip a small glass of freshly-squeezed, or even frozen, fruit juice, such as orange or grapefruit. Within three minutes, the fructose in the juice should raise your blood sugar level to the point where your craving has almost disappeared.

105

•*Step 2.*

Use the STOP technique to halt the addiction in its tracks. Snap the rubber band on your wrist (see FF#2-A). Then call out "Stop," or say it silently if others are present. Next, while you relax, take six deep, slow breaths. Each time you exhale, repeat the word "Stop."

This behavioral strategy, designed to change the way you feel by the way you act, gives you time to pause and recognize the mistake you are about to make. If you feel at all guilty or uncomfortable, it is usually an indication that you are about to indulge in an energy-robbing addiction.

•*Step 3.*

Experience your craving. Close your eyes and note exactly where in your body the craving is located. Place your awareness on this spot and experience the craving. What does the craving feel like? What color, shape and texture does it have? What does it remind you of? (Example: "The craving is located in my solar plexus. It feels like a lead weight dragging me down and draining my energy. It is gray in color and I sense that it is smooth and round.")

Great! Now, still keeping your eyes closed, let your mind experience all this for 30 to 60 seconds. Next, use your imagination to project the heavy, gray, smooth sphere to a point about ten feet in front of you. Visualize it out there in space. Then expand it to ten times its size. Experience that.

Now fill it with water. How much water will it hold? Experience it. Next, picture the water running out.

This time, shrink the heavy gray sphere down to one-tenth its original size. Visualize it as small as a marble. Experience it once more. Fill it with water again and see how much it holds.

Experience that. Then empty the sphere. Expand it back to its original size. Experience it again. Finally, place it back in your body.

Ask yourself again what you are experiencing. Most people find that their craving has disappeared entirely. And chances are good that it will not bother them again for at least an hour.

•*Step 4.*

To ensure that your blood sugar level remains stable, eat a complex carbohydrate snack such as a bowl of cereal or vegetable soup as soon as possible.

CAFFEINE—A LEGAL SHOT OF SPEED

A cup of coffee gives you a legal dose of speed that quickly boosts mental alertness and performance. Just as swiftly, it releases stress hormones that liberate glycogen from the liver to fill the muscles with immediate energy.

Caffeine does indeed arouse the mind and get it racing— but only for a brief while. It does so by making the brain more sensitive to the neurotransmitter norepinephrine. But in under an hour, supplies run low and a person feels mentally slow and fatigued once more.

Endurance athletes by the hundreds also rely on caffeine to start the liver releasing glycogen immediately instead of 15 or 20 minutes into a race. Studies show, however, that this strategy works best only for people who are not habitual users of caffeine. Extensive research has demonstrated that caffeine does improve performance in people who are not accustomed to drinking caffeine regularly. And this superior performance will last throughout a race provided a cup of coffee is consumed at regular intervals.

A single cup will also help a chronic coffee user to release glycogen at the beginning of a race. But a second cup will cause a decline in energy and lead to early fatigue. No amount of additional coffee will increase energy. Nor does caffeine enhance stamina by causing the body to burn fat for energy, as was once thought.

HOW MUCH COFFEE CAN YOU SAFELY CONSUME?

Although some people can drink one or two cups of coffee a day without serious energy loss, others experience an afternoon letdown from just one cup at breakfast. Higher doses can over-stimulate and stress the nervous system, heighten anxiety, and cause restlessness, insomnia and wide mood swings. A study at Stanford University Medical School found that students who consumed five or more cups of coffee a day soon established a dependency. They experienced withdrawal symptoms on awakening and they needed a new fix to begin the day.

Pharmacologists consider that 260 mg of caffeine consumed over a short period is a fairly high dose while 500 mg per day is an equally heavy intake. Addiction becomes almost inevitable when these levels are maintained.

A six-ounce cup of brewed coffee contains an average 80

to 100 mg of caffeine while a strong cup can contain 150 to 180 mg. Percolated coffee averages 110 mg per cup, instant coffee 70 to 80, black tea 40 to 60, cocoa 50 and a 12-ounce caffeinated soda 32 to 65 mg. Chocolate is another source of caffeine, as are several popular brands of over-the-counter painkilling medications.

From an energy-conservation point of view, caffeine is obviously something we'd all be better off without. The action step below describes how to eliminate it for good.

•FATIGUE FIGHTER #6: Stop Caffeine from Draining Your Energy

Caffeine dependence and its associated withdrawal symptoms are one of the most common causes of chronic fatigue.

If a single cup makes you feel tense, wired-up, hyper-alert, or even agitated, you may be unusually sensitive to caffeine. And if, when you eliminate caffeine, you develop a mild headache and feel tired or drowsy, then caffeine may well be contributing to your chronic fatigue.

Fortunately, caffeine is a comparatively mild drug and the following steps are designed to provide a painless withdrawal.

•Step 1.

For one week, replace each five-ounce cup of coffee that you normally drink with half a cupful.

•Step 2.

For the second week, replace each half cup of coffee you have been drinking with a full cup of medium-strength black tea.

109

•*Step 3.*

For the third week, replace the last cup of tea of the day with a cup of herb tea or with fruit juice cut with water or with a sports drink.

•*Step 4.*

For the fourth week, again replace what has become the last cup of tea of the day with a cup of herb tea, or fruit juice and water, or a sports drink.

Continue with the same program until you are no longer drinking any black tea. At this point, you should be caffeine-free.

If at any time, you experience a craving for coffee, practice the technique in FF#5. Alternatively, instead of drinking caffeine, take a short, brisk walk or eat some vegetable sticks or a piece of fruit or take a brisk shower—or do all of these.

To help you stay off caffeine, avoid all foods high in refined carbohydrates, including processed and manufactured foods, baked goods, jams, jellies, pastries, ice cream, candies and all foods containing significant amounts of sugar, honey, molasses or other sweeteners. Build your meals instead around vegetables, whole grains and legumes. These foods maintain the blood sugar at a stable level, thus preventing the energy drop in response to which we turn to caffeine.

NICOTINE—AN INSIDIOUS DESTROYER OF ENERGY AND LIFE

Cigarette smoking is a suicidal, health-wrecking habit that directly suppresses energy, intensifies chronic tiredness and virtually guarantees a premature one-way trip to Forest Lawn.

Not only are smokers likely to be sick and to experience more stress than nonsmokers, but they ignore their health more often and report much greater dissatisfaction with their lives. According to a study by the Imperial Cancer Research Center of the United Kingdom (reported in the May 23, 1992 issue of *Lancet*), cigarette smoking kills one of every five persons in all Western industrial nations. In the U.S., where one person in four still smokes, this means that 80 percent of all Americans who smoke will die from the effects of cigarette smoking.

Most people smoke because nicotine intensifies their arousal and alertness and creates a pleasurable "high" while subduing most feelings of pain and anxiety. Curiously, these are exactly the same reactions that follow a session of aerobic exercise. Take a brisk walk for half an hour and you also can experience heightened arousal and alertness, a pleasant endorphin "high" and a disappearance of almost all pain and anxiety. Moreover, the positive benefits of walking last the remainder of the day, while those from nicotine seldom endure for more than 45 minutes.

That's because cigarettes are the most addictive of all adrenal stimulants. The adrenal glands of most smokers are so chronically fatigued and exhausted that it may be necessary to chain smoke to keep them stimulated.

Almost everyone is aware that smoking is a major cause of heart disease, stroke, cancer, diabetes and renal disease. Smoking also intensifies fatigue by creating serious sleep difficulties. And it heightens anxiety and depression.

111

SMOKING MUST GO

None of us can hope to successfully restore our energy until we quit smoking for good. Recent studies have also demonstrated that major health risks—including energy loss—can also arise from passive smoking (inhaling smoke from another person's cigarette).

For most smokers, there is no time to lose. The longer you have smoked, the more likely your adrenals are to be fatigued or exhausted, and the greater the risk to your health.

Although a complete review of stop-smoking techniques is beyond the scope of this book, I recommend using FFs#2 and 2-A to help yourself quit. As you may recall, these action-steps utilize immediate feedback to reinforce your win-power and determination to remain a nonsmoker.

And I guarantee that when you quit smoking, feedback will be swift and dramatic. Within hours, almost every former smoker experiences incredible relief. Coughing ceases. Sleep improves. The natural ability to taste and smell quickly return. And within days, your energy level will begin to soar.

QUITTING ON YOUR OWN IS BEST

Many people delay quitting in order to join a stop-smoking group. But motivational studies show that the success rate of those who quit on their own is twice that of those who join a group.

A recent study by Dr. Michael C. Fiore of the University of Wisconsin found that smokers who quit cold turkey on their own succeed twice as often as those who enroll in a group. However, Dr. Fiore acknowledges that some really heavy smokers could benefit from smoking cessation programs.

Quit-smoking groups range from inexpensive workshops run by nonprofit groups like the American Cancer Society, American Lung Association and the Seventh Day Adventists to others operated by for-profit organizations. A recent survey found that both types had an equal success rate. Aversion therapy (see FF#2-A), under the supervision of a professional behavioral therapist, is another option. Still another effective method is a strongly-worded order from your doctor commanding you to stop smoking now.

AIDS FOR KICKING THE SMOKING HABIT

Among stop-smoking aids are nicotine chewing gum and nicotine patches. Both are designed to permit painless withdrawal by releasing nicotine into the bloodstream at a gradually decreasing rate. The gum is chewed into a wad and placed in the cheek to allow the nicotine to be absorbed through the mucous membrane lining the mouth. Also available are transdermal nicotine patches which deliver a low level of nicotine through the skin. Since either may interact with certain drugs, they should be used only under medical supervision.

Again, since caffeine exacerbates nicotine withdrawal symptoms, most authorities recommend that you withdraw from caffeine either before, or at the same time as, you quit smoking. Most of us are also aware by now that switching to low tar and low-yield cigarettes doesn't help. Surveys show that such strategies merely increase the craving for more and more cigarettes.

Nor should you allow fear of weight gain to deter you

113

from ceasing to smoke. To equal the health risks of smoking, a person would have to be 120 pounds overweight. Even if weight gain does occur after smoking, it need only be temporary.

•FATIGUE FIGHTER #7: How to Stop Smoking by the Five-Minute Method

This painless smoking withdrawal plan is based on research which found that smokers tend to light up most under two conditions: when their blood sugar is low and when they begin to feel drowsy after a heavy meal.

The principle of the program is to add five minutes to each interval between cigarettes (or pipes or cigars). You begin with a one-hour interval. Your next cigarette is due one hour and five minutes later. The next will be due one hour and ten minutes later. And so on. Each interval becomes five minutes longer than the previous interval.

You also make a commitment not to smoke for one hour after waking up, not to smoke for one hour before bedtime, and not to smoke for one hour after finishing any meal.

Between now and starting time, write out a list of reasons why you wish to stop smoking. (Examples: "To rid myself of smoker's cough and phlegm in my lungs; to be able to smell and taste once more; to restore my energy and overcome fatigue; to rid myself of bad breath; and to save myself from dying of heart disease or cancer.")

Also before beginning, lay in a stock of fruit juices, chewing gum, plain popcorn, and dried fruits—virtually any healthy non-stimulant you can think of to replace the satisfaction of a cigarette. You will also need two packs of the brand of cigarettes you hate the most.

Set a date to begin this program within a week. Friday is the ideal day to start since it gives you the second and third days at home away from job stress. Once you begin, avoid any commitments for the following two weeks that might increase your stress. That includes staying away from any social engagements in which you might be pressured into drinking alcohol or coffee or eating sweets. You should also eliminate all other refined carbohydrates from your diet, reduce the fat and animal protein and increase complex carbohydrates (FF#9 and 11).

On starting day, and each day thereafter, psych yourself up with Win-Power (FF#2) as soon as you wake up. Then read the list of reasons why you wish to quit. Whenever you feel like smoking, use the Stop Technique (FF#2-A) and read the list of reasons why you wish to stop smoking. Whenever you feel the urge to smoke, practice the steps in FF#5.

After getting out of bed on your first day, throw away your remaining cigarettes together with ashtrays, lighters and other smoking paraphernalia. From now on you may smoke only the brand of cigarettes you hate the most and only at the permissible intervals.

Your first day's program will probably look like this:

7:00 a.m.	get up
8-8:30	breakfast
9:30	first cigarette
10:35	second cigarette
11:45	third cigarette
12:30-1 p.m.	lunch
2:00	fourth cigarette
3:15	fifth cigarette
4:35	sixth cigarette
6:00	seventh cigarette

115

7-7:30	dinner
8:30	eighth cigarette
10:30	bedtime

Under the Five-Minute Plan, eight cigarettes is about the maximum you can squeeze into the first day. Should you wake up during the night craving a cigarette, use the Stop Technique and feel free to enjoy unlimited snacks (complex carbohydrates only, of course). Cigarette smoking is so life-threatening that almost anything you can do to help break it is permissible. For instance, don't worry about putting on weight. Research shows that it is only temporary. And always bear in mind that the best substitute for a cigarette is a brisk half-hour walk (or a swim, bicycle ride or tennis game). Any type of rhythmic exercise will help break dependence on nicotine and will also improve your sleep.

Whenever you have a few moments to spare, relax and use FF#18 to visualize yourself as a non-smoker setting out on a wonderful new life with unlimited energy and stamina. Picture yourself able to taste and smell again. See yourself enjoying a large salad of fresh garden vegetables without any dressing and experience the honest taste of each vegetable in the bowl.

Make mental pictures of your lungs changing from tar-blackened air sacs into pink, healthy organs. See yourself striding briskly along a beach with the salty tang of surf in your nostrils and the cries of swooping gulls overhead. Experience yourself waking up fully refreshed and filled with zip and vigor every morning for the rest of your life.

Visualize goals which assume you are already a non-smoker. Picture yourself walking up mountain trails as you inhale lungfuls of cool, fresh air. Recognize that by cutting

116

out smoking you will soon feel and act as though you were ten years younger. Think about spending your next vacation walking in the Rockies or trekking in the Himalayas.

By the sixth morning, the interval between cigarettes will have grown to two hours and forty minutes and your day's smoking schedule should look something like this.

7:00 a.m.	get up
8-8:30	breakfast
9:30	first cigarette
12:10 p.m.	second cigarette
12:30-1	lunch
2:00	third cigarette
4:45	fourth cigarette
7-7:30	dinner
8:30	fifth cigarette
10:30	bedtime

By now, you are smoking so few cigarettes, and at such long intervals, that on the seventh morning, you can easily stop smoking altogether. During the five following nicotine-free days continue to use all of the anti-smoking techniques and aids to offset any urge to smoke.

Positive feedback should be abundant by now. Your sleep pattern should have improved. Your fatigue should have diminished and your energy should have doubled. And you will be enjoying life for the first time since you began to smoke regularly.

By the twelfth day you can begin to let go of the snacks and beverages that helped you break the cigarette habit. At this point, you should have totally broken all physical dependence on nicotine.

117

ALCOHOL—A MAJOR RISK FACTOR FOR CHRONIC TIREDNESS

The health risks of regular, long-term alcohol consumption are too well known to need repeating. Steady drinking is a major risk factor for cancer, hypertension and stroke and it blocks absorption of many nutrients essential to proper functioning of the energy mechanism. Alcohol also intensifies fatigue by interfering with sleep and by increasing dehydration. It has all the drawbacks of other refined carbohydrates. And since it cannot be stored as glycogen, alcohol is not even a good source of energy.

Most authorities believe that—except for pregnant women and people with liver damage—a maximum of two drinks per day will not seriously impair the energy mechanism. (A drink is usually defined as an eight or 12 ounce can of beer, a three to four ounce glass of wine, or an ounce of distilled spirits.) But a steady consumption of even one or two drinks per day may lead to chronic tiredness in alcohol-sensitive individuals.

In view of these facts, anyone who is serious about beating chronic tiredness is strongly advised to eliminate alcohol altogether, at least until they are back in balance. This is especially true if you are below average in weight. While two drinks a day might not seriously affect a 220 pound man, they could play havoc with the energy mechanism of a 110 pound woman.

118

•FATIGUE FIGHTER #8: Ending Alcohol-Induced Chronic Tiredness Caused by Mildly Habitual Dependence

Let's assume you have become habitually dependent on drinking four beers, or other drinks, each evening after work. You feel that these drinks are your reward for getting through the day. Assuming that you do not consume additional alcohol during the day, you can easily break dependence on this amount of alcohol and can end all alcohol-induced chronic tiredness.

Begin by using FFs#1 and 2 to boost your motivation to act now. Don't permit anything to delay or postpone your determination to end the alcohol habit now and forever. Otherwise, what may still be a mild dependency may become a hard-to-break addiction.

Beginning this evening, you will taper off alcohol consumption by taking one drink less per day. This evening, you will take three drinks, tomorrow two drinks and the next evening one drink and after that, no drinks at all.

Shortly before taking your first evening drink, prepare all four of your usual drinks and place them in front of you. This means you will be sitting down facing four cans or glasses of beer, wine or liquor.

At this point, begin to use a well-known behavioral therapy technique (described in full in FF#2-A: Using Aversion Therapy to Stop Energy-Depleting Addictions).

Take one drink in your hand, place it close to your lips, then replace it untouched on the table. Snap the rubber band on your wrist and use the Stop Technique (described

119

in FF#2-A). Call out, "Stop!" Then, while you relax, take six slow, deep breaths. Each time you exhale, repeat the word, "Stop!"

This strategy gives you time to pause and recognize your mistake. If you feel at all uncomfortable or guilty, this is a strong indication that you are about to indulge in an energy-robbing addiction.

In under one minute, this simple procedure will empower you to stop seeing yourself as hopelessly addicted to the beer (or wine or liquor). Instead of being unable to stop yourself from drinking the beer, you will swiftly realize that you are a powerful person and that you have complete control over your life, your health and your energy level.

So reinforce your empowerment by picking up your beer glass again and affirming, "I am a powerful person. I have unlimited self-discipline and self-control. I choose to not drink this beer tonight nor on any night in future. I have the ability to stop drinking beer completely. And I rejoice in the knowledge that I am no longer addicted to any form of alcohol."

Replace the drink on the table. Then repeat this exercise nine more times, each time replacing the drink untouched on the table.

As soon as you complete this routine, get up and pour the drink down the kitchen sink. As you do, experience gratitude for having not drunk it. Place the remaining three drinks in the refrigerator. You may then consume the three drinks provided they are spread over the same time period in which you habitually consume four drinks.

This gradual tapering-off method should prevent any serious withdrawal discomfort. Remind yourself often that you will shortly become a non-drinker and anticipate how good it will feel to have more energy and to sleep more soundly.

Next evening, repeat the entire routine again. Place the same four drinks on the table. But this time, repeat the technique ten times with the first drink and ten more times with the second drink.

You will then throw away both drinks and you will consume the remaining two drinks spread over your usual drinking period.

On the third evening, stack four drinks on the table and go through the behavioral therapy routine on each of three drinks. Throw these three drinks away and consume only one drink spread over your habitual drinking period.

To fill any vacuum previously filled by the drinks, chew gum or eat a snack of any complex carbohydrate food such as fruit, vegetable sticks, plain air-popped popcorn or a whole wheat bread sandwich. Never use caffeine or sugar to fill the gap. A brisk daily walk or other rhythmic exercise will provide immediate feedback in the shape of improved energy, better sleep and a more cheerful mood.

On the fourth evening, place all four drinks on the table. Use the behavioral therapy technique on each of the four. Then throw away all four drinks. Replace the alcohol with a glass of fruit juice cut with water, a glass of warm skim milk or with a sports drink or any other beverage that is free of alcohol, caffeine and sugar.

Repeat the same routine with each of the four drinks on the fifth, sixth and seventh evenings. Experience deep gratitude as you pour each drink down the drain.

That should do it! By now, you should have broken both physical and psychological dependence on alcohol. Incidentally, you can use this same action-step to break dependence on caffeine, nicotine or just about anything else.

IF YOU FALL OFF THE WAGON

Whichever addiction you're trying to break, if you do happen to "fall off the wagon," use aversion therapy to get back on track right away. Drinking one cup of coffee or smoking one cigarette while you're trying to quit is no reason to change your long-term goals. That is, provided you stop right there and get back on the wagon immediately. FF#2-A gives full instructions for using aversion therapy to get back on track.

CHAPTER EIGHT

Foods That Fight Fatigue

Popeye was right. Plant foods have much more readily available energy than meat or dairy products. In the athletic world, performance levels are so high nowadays that only a meatless diet can provide the energy for champions to win. Moreover, every major health advisory agency is telling us that these same high energy plant foods can dramatically lower our risk of ever getting heart disease, cancer, diabetes and other common killer diseases.

These foods that provide both high energy and health in a single package are fresh fruits, vegetables, legumes, whole grains and seeds. All grow on plants and are known to nutritionists as *complex carbohydrates*.

To eat for high energy, we need to know that the body prefers to obtain its energy from carbohydrate foods. Fats are the body's second choice energy foods. And the body would prefer not to use protein for energy at all.

Since man evolved as a plant-eating higher primate, our genes have given us a digestive system designed to swiftly liberate energy from plant foods, that is, from carbohydrates. While exercising, for example, we can begin drawing on energy from many plant foods within 30 minutes of eating, or even less. By comparison, it may take eight hours or more to digest fat to the point where its energy becomes available. Even then, the body will not use fat if energy from carbohydrates can be drawn on instead.

But there are "good" and "bad" carbohydrates. The good carbohydrates, called complex carbohydrates, consist of plant foods still in the original state in which they grew. This means they are still whole and unfragmented and have not been devitalized by processing or manufacturing.

Coarse milling, such as stone ground milling, is permissible to reduce whole grains into flour or oats into oatmeal. But the whole grain flour or oatmeal still retains most of its original fiber and nutrients.

BAD CARBOHYDRATES

Bad carbohydrates are called simple or refined carbohydrates. They started out as unprocessed wheat, sugar or rice. But the millers and the food industry discovered they could maximize profits by refining these complex carbohydrates into white flour, white sugar and white rice. By transforming these natural foods into unnatural refined carbohydrates, they stripped virtually all the fiber and other nutrients from the white flour and white sugar, leaving little more than empty calories. While white rice isn't quite as depleted, it should never be eaten when brown rice is available.

Certainly, refined carbohydrates are still high in energy. But because their cell walls have been destroyed by milling, their starches and sugars are swiftly released and transformed into glucose which pours into the bloodstream in a sudden flush. Chapter 4 explains the mechanisms by which this flood of glucose overwhelms the ability of the pancreas to secrete insulin. Instead of turning the surplus glucose into glycogen, to be stored in the liver and muscles for future use, the rush of glucose simply drives up the blood sugar level. In most people, the glucose is soon used up. And without glycogen reserves to draw on, the blood sugar level then plummets. The result is low blood sugar, which is the same as feeling drained of energy.

Without delving further into the chemistry of foods, it should be obvious that, besides failing to deliver the nutrients the body requires, refined carbohydrates are not the foods the body needs to fight fatigue. Yet more than one-fifth of all foods eaten by the average American consist of refined carbohydrates.

GOOD CARBOHYDRATES

Complex carbohydrates, by contrast, are composed of living cells, each enclosed by a cellulose wall. Since it takes time for the cellulose to break down, the sugars and starches in complex carbohydrates are released at a stable rate. This provides the muscles with a slow-burning fuel. The roller-coaster blood sugar levels associated with refined carbohydrates never occur. Diabetes is rare. The discarded cellulose

125

supplies the digestive system with badly-needed fiber. And each complex carbohydrate food is also a rich source of vitamins and minerals.

The focus of most of the dietary advice published by such organizations as the American Heart Association, the American Cancer Society, the Framingham Heart Study and the National Academy of Sciences is to reduce by half or more our daily intake of calories from fat and animal protein and to at least double our intake of calories from vegetables, fruits, whole grains and legumes. That's because a high fat diet has been clearly identified as a primary cause of heart disease and stroke, hypertension, diabetes, obesity and cancer of the breast, colon and prostate.

Besides supplying calories to power the brain and muscles, complex carbohydrates help prevent a variety of life-threatening diseases. For instance, broccoli, brussel sprouts, cauliflower, peas, beans and seeds all contain protease inhibitors which protect against cancer. All yellow-orange fruits and vegetables, and dark green leafy vegetables, are rich in beta-carotene, an anti-oxidant that also prevents cancer and heart disease.

DIETARY BLUEPRINT FOR ENERGY AND HEALTH

According to government and other health advisory agencies, we should eat two to four servings of fruit, three to five servings of vegetables and six to eleven servings of whole grains each day. Yet a recent survey by a U.S. government agency revealed that fewer than nine percent of Americans ate a minimum of two servings of fruit and three servings of vegetables daily.

The typical American diet obtains only 42 percent of calories from carbohydrates (largely refined) while 39 percent is from fat (much of it dangerous saturated fat), and 19 percent is derived from protein (mostly obtained from meat and dairy products). Nutritionists describe this as a 42-39-19 diet.

Not only is this diet low in energy but it supplies barely one-third of the body's daily fiber needs. Complex carbohydrates, especially grains, contain large amounts of both soluble and insoluble fiber. Soluble fiber helps normalize blood sugar and lower elevated cholesterol while insoluble fiber reduces risk of colon cancer. Most authorities recommend that we consume 25 to 35 grams of fiber daily. A high-energy complex carbohydrate diet could easily provide 40 grams of health-enhancing fiber per day.

WHY FAT IS A POOR FUEL

Only limited energy is derived from fat. As reserves of glycogen are gradually drawn down while walking, for example, the body turns to fat as a second choice fuel. After walking for one hour, we may be drawing 85 percent of our energy from glucose (carbohydrate fuel) and 15 percent from fat. After walking for two hours, the ratio may have changed to 75 percent from glucose and 25 percent from fat. But speed up your pace and the body immediately ceases to use fat and begins to burn glucose exclusively.

Should we really run low on glucose and glycogen, and the body is forced to burn fat for energy, it produces a toxic by-product called ketones. To flush out the ketones requires so much water that a person may become dehydrated and fatigued.

Any diet in which 35 to 40 percent of calories are derived from fat is classified as a high-fat diet. A low-fat diet derives 20 percent or less of calories from fat. And a very low-fat diet derives ten percent or less of calories from fat. Most Americans eat a high-fat diet.

Although most health advisory agencies advise the American public to reduce fat intake to 30 percent of calories or less, most research shows that heart disease and cancer rates don't begin to improve significantly until the fat content of the diet is cut to 20 percent or less.

Virtually all of us could boost our intake of readily available energy by reducing fat intake to 20 percent of calories or less. This enables us to replace the fat with a variety of complex carbohydrates. This simple strategy changes the standard 42-39-19 American diet into a much improved 61-20-19 formula.

WHY PROTEIN FAILS TO POWER THE MUSCLES

Protein consists of 22 amino acids which, in a variety of combinations, form the tissues, cells, bones, nerves, muscles and organs of the body. Since our bodies can synthesize only 13 amino acids, the remaining nine—called essential amino acids (EAAs)—must be obtained directly from the diet. Virtually all foods of animal origin— including meat, fish, poultry, eggs and dairy products—supply all nine EAAs. But no single plant food contains whole protein.

Nevertheless, by eating a variety of vegetables, grains and beans each day, a plant-based diet can easily meet our protein needs. Those amino acids lacking in one plant food are supplied by another. Complementing almost any whole grain with a legume results in complete protein. In fact, a combination of rice and beans, or corn and beans, or whole grain bread and peanut butter results in protein equal in quality to any obtainable from eggs, meat or dairy products. Anyone who eats a variety of vegetables, grains and legumes each day can depend on having an ample supply of whole protein without needing to eat any animal-derived foods.

This means that we can obtain at least half, or even all, of our protein from high-energy complex carbohydrates. We can thus obtain protein plus energy, not merely protein plus fat, as is the case with most meat and dairy products. Considering that animal protein usually comes together with fat, and has been linked to heart disease, cancer and most other degenerative diseases, getting our protein from complex carbohydrates can be a giant step towards improved energy and better health.

That 61-20-19 formula might optimally become 65-15-20. By making all of the carbohydrates complex, we would have a true "hi-carb" diet.

EATING TO WIN—WITH A HI-CARB DIET

Most endurance athletes—those who walk, run, bicycle, swim or ski long distances—know from experience that only a hi-carb diet can supply the edge they need to win. Which is why, throughout the world, millions of athletes and other active people rely on a hi-carb diet to supply their energy needs.

129

Meanwhile, a "low-carb" diet, implying a diet low in complex carbohydrates, (and therefore high in refined carbohydrates, fat and animal protein) has proved to be a common cause of chronic tiredness and even biochemically-induced depression. When associated with a sedentary lifestyle, a low-carb diet almost invariably leads to some degree of chronic tiredness coupled with mediocre health.

You can change all that by switching from a low-carb to a hi-carb diet. The following Fatigue Fighters are designed to help you make the switch.

•FATIGUE FIGHTER #9: Replace Excessive Dietary Fat with High-Energy Foods

Not only is fat a second class muscle fuel but the excessive amounts eaten by most Americans prevents people from eating the high-energy complex carbohydrates they really need.

To pep up your energy resources, you must cut fat intake from the American average of 39 percent of calories to 20 percent or less. Most manufacturers list the fat content of foods by weight. But nutritionists find it more meaningful to measure the fat, protein and carbohydrate content of foods as a percentage of total calories. A calorie is a measure of the heat, or energy, liberated from a food when it is transformed by the muscles into mechanical energy. One gram of either carbohydrate or protein contains four calories, while one gram of fat contains nine calories.

So how does a meal look if 20 percent of its calories are derived from fat?

For the average man to cut fat intake from 40 to 20

130

percent of calories means cutting out approximately 56 grams of fat per day. That is equivalent to two ounces or two tablespoons. But only sticks of butter or margarine, or bottled oils, can be measured in spoonfuls. The rest must be estimated.

FINDING THE FAT CONTENT OF PROCESSED FOODS

However, a simple formula exists by which we can calculate the exact percentage of fat calories in any packaged food that carries a nutrition label. For example, most processed foods carry a label listing the number of grams of fat and the total calories per serving.

After May 1994, all packaged foods must bear a label giving these amounts plus the weight of total fat, saturated fat, cholesterol, sodium, carbohydrates, sugars, dietary fiber and protein. Then, based on a recommended daily diet of 2,000 calories, including 65 grams of fat, the label will show the percentage of each of these nutritional factors in a single serving. Also, serving sizes will be standardized. However, the new labels still do not give the percentage of calories from fat.

Nonetheless, both old and new labels list the number of grams of total fat and the number of calories per serving. From these two factors, the following formula gives the percentage of calories from fat.

Let's say that a tablespoon of peanut butter has a fat content of 7.2 grams and contains 86 calories.

Step 1: multiply the number of grams per serving by nine,

the number of calories in each gram of fat. (Example: 7.2 × 9 = 64.8)

Step 2: divide the answer to Step 1 by the number of calories per serving. (Example: 64.8 ÷ 86 = .753)

Step 3: multiply the answer to Step 2 by 100. (Example: .753 × 100 = 75.3)

The formula shows that the peanut butter has a fat content of 75 percent, meaning that 75 percent of calories are from fat.

Another example: a can of soup has three grams of fat and 65 calories per serving. The calculation is:

3 × 9 = 27 ÷ 65 = .41 × 100 = 41

Thus 41 percent of calories in this soup is from fat.

Regardless of serving size, the formula works on any food for which nutritional information is given. Applying the formula to milk may give us a nasty jolt. Although whole milk is only four percent fat by weight, most of the milk consists of water which has no nutritional value. When we subtract the water, the formula reveals that the fat content of the remaining milk solids averages 48 percent. Even two percent milk derives some 38 percent of calories from fat, while one percent milk has 18 percent fat calories. These are hardly low fat levels.

The formula also reveals a different story to claims such as "95 percent fat-free," which still may be seen on canned meats and other foods until May 1994. The label correctly implies that the fat content is 5 percent *by weight*. But the formula shows that the percentage of calories from fat is 10.6 percent—more than double that claimed on the label.

If you must eat processed foods, it's a good idea to limit them to foods which derive only 20 percent of calories, or less, from fat.

FINE TUNE YOUR FAT INTAKE

Let's say we're following a 70-15-15 diet, meaning 70 percent of calories is from carbohydrates, 15 percent is from fat and 15 percent from protein. Whether by weight or volume, a plate of food based on this formula will contain approximately 68 percent carbohydrates, 9 percent fat, and 23 percent protein. The fat content is small in size or weight but each gram of fat contains more than twice as many calories (9) as each gram of carbohydrate or protein (4). Thus small quantities of fat can represent a large percentage of the calories in any meal.

This example demonstrates why fat must be ruthlessly cut from the diet, not merely because it impedes the energy mechanism but because it is a major risk factor for heart disease, cancer and most other degenerative diseases.

Most of us have read about the various kinds of fat. Saturated fats, found mostly in meats, dairy products, and tropical oils, are the most potent promoters of artery blockage in existence. Even polyunsaturated fats, such as corn, safflower or sunflower seed oils, are considered quite hazardous nowadays. When used for cooking at high temperatures, they release highly reactive free radicals that can also block arteries and cause cancer and other diseases.

Monounsaturated fats, such as olive or canola oils, are probably the least dangerous fats as far as cancer and heart disease are concerned, yet they still derive 100 percent of their calories from fat. Partially-hydrogenated vegetable oils are vegetable oils made more dangerous through processing. They are found in virtually every type of commercial baked goods, breads and processed foods, and are the main component of margarine.

133

Obviously, we should try to minimize all saturated, poly-unsaturated and partially-hydrogenated vegetable oils in our diet. However, in selecting an oil for cooking, baking, or for salads, olive and canola oils are considered least harmful.

Don't be afraid of cutting out too much fat. Except for tiny amounts of linoleic and linolenic fatty acids, the body can synthesize all other fats it needs from carbohydrates. Few of us need to eat more fat and certainly not as an energy source. The almost universal advice of the preventive medicine school, and many other nutritionists and cardiologists, is to limit fat intake to a maximum of 20 percent of calories (a low-fat diet) or to 10 to 15 percent of calories (a very low-fat diet) if you are recovering from or at risk for heart disease or cancer.

Despite this and other advice to lower fat, the average American continues to eat 66 pounds of fats and oils per year, 11 gallons of ice cream, 79 pounds of beef and 261 eggs. Many people eat much more.

A ROGUE'S GALLERY OF HIGH-FAT FOODS

Among common foods with the highest fat content are: pastries, beef, butter, candy, cheese, cheeseburgers, chocolate, cream cheese, cured and processed meats, salad dressings, egg yolks, fast foods, fried foods, frozen dinners, granola bars, ice cream, lamb, margarine, mayonnaise, milk (whole and low-fat), nuts, olives, organ meats, peanut butter, pizza, popcorn (commercial), pork, potato chips, croissants, cream sauces, sausage and luncheon meat, sour cream, and whipped toppings.

Light versions of some of these foods may be an improvement, but not always.

If this list contains some of your favorite foods, you can find consolation in learning that most people who switch to a hi-carb diet discover a wealth of new gustatory pleasures. Complex carbohydrates offer unlimited opportunities for gourmet cooking. For instance, you can draw on the great culinary traditions of countries like Italy, India, China and Japan where people live more active lives, and have higher energy levels, than in the U.S. They also have dramatically lower rates of heart disease and stroke.

It's also quite possible to reduce the amount of fat in almost any standard recipe by 50 to 66 percent without any reduction of eating pleasure. To cut fat, try sauteeing in water or fruit juice; use only egg whites and discard the yolks; replace oil in recipes with fruit concentrates; and use plain nonfat yogurt in place of sour cream, regular mayonnaise, and salad dressings.

MAKING HEALTHY FOODS UNHEALTHY

We also tend to transform healthy hi-carb foods like a potato, or a slice of bread, into high-fat foods by slathering them with butter, sour cream or mayonnaise. A plain baked potato has only 100 calories and almost zero fat. But when we plaster it with sour cream, it suddenly contains 300 calories and if we fry it, it contains 500 calories. Yet originally, it was a healthful complex carbohydrate food. All too often, it's what we put on healthful foods that makes them hazardous to health. Thus when, in this book, I say "a potato" or "a slice of bread" I mean exactly that, not a potato loaded with butter and cream nor a slice of bread layered with mayonnaise.

For breakfast, oatmeal and fresh fruits soon become more

135

enjoyable than ham and eggs. Lunch can include vegetable soup and a large raw vegetable salad with a dressing of plain nonfat yogurt. Dinner can focus on entrees of vegetables, baked potatoes, and tasty soups, stews, casseroles and low-fat grain-based dishes. Herbs and spices can replace high fat sauces, gravies, oils, butter or cream. And fresh fruits can replace desserts loaded with fat and refined carbohydrates.

After a few days of low-fat eating, most people feel so good that it never occurs to them to feel restricted or deprived.

Eating fish is often touted as safer than eating meat, eggs, poultry or dairy products. But eating beans and whole grains instead provides less cholesterol and more energy.

If you must eat meat or poultry, be sure to remove the skin from chicken and all visible fat from meat. Turkey has less fat than chicken. And chicken thighs, wings and backs have much more fat than the breast. If you buy ground chicken or turkey meat, make sure it is labelled "skinless." Pork, beef and lamb are generally high in fat. But top round steak has the lowest fat content of any meat.

As you've probably noticed, virtually all animal foods high in fat are also high in protein. And most are equally high in cholesterol. Thus cutting back on fat also helps reduce our intake of dietary cholesterol and animal protein—two things that most of us eat to excess.

•FATIGUE FIGHTER #10: Replace These Counterfeit Foods with Energy-Filled Complex Carbohydrates

Nutritionally-depleted refined carbohydrates are a significant cause of chronic tiredness as well as other energy-sapping dysfunctions. The following refined carbohydrate foods and beverages should be swiftly and permanently phased out of the diet.

Alcohol, soft drinks, candy, chewing gum, chocolate, white flour and white sugar, and almost all sweeteners, are refined carbohydrates, including brown sugar, honey, maple syrup and molasses. Other food products high in refined carbohydrates include white bread, pies, pastries, ice cream, flour tortillas, cakes, cookies, baked goods, white flour bagels and pita bread, and junk food, as well as many manufactured and processed foods.

Within an hour of eating a meal high in refined carbohydrates, many people experience mood swings, a decrease in memory, anxiety, mild depression and fatigue. If eaten late in the evening, sleeplessness may occur.

•FATIGUE FIGHTER #11: Power Foods—Fifty Foods with the Highest Readily-Available Energy

Listed below are the 50 foods believed to contain the highest amounts of readily-available carbohydrate energy. Almost all are complex carbohydrates. High in fiber and other essential nutrients, their inclusion in your diet should have an immediate beneficial effect. We recommend that you eat them in place of the fat and refined carbohydrates eliminated by Fatigue Fighters #9 and #10.

*FRUITS: apricots, avocados, bananas, canteloupes, melons (all types), papaya, peaches, pineapples.

*LEGUMES: azuki beans, black beans, black-eyed peas, garbanzo beans (chick peas), great northern beans, kidney beans, lentils, lima beans, navy beans, peas—all types, soybeans, tempeh, tofu.

137

*TUBERS: beets, carrots, jicama, parsnips, potatoes, ruta-
bagas, sweet potatoes, turnips, yams.

*VEGETABLES: cucumbers, kohlrabi, pumpkin, squash—
all types.

*WHOLE GRAINS: barley, bran muffins, bread—whole
grain, bulgur wheat, corn, cornmeal (unrefined), corn tortillas, cracked wheat, granola, grits, hominy, kasha, millet,
muesli, oat bran, oatmeal, pasta (whole grain), rice (whole
grain, brown), rye, rye flour, shredded wheat, sprouted grains
bread, sunflower seeds, triticale, wheat, whole wheat bread
and bagels, whole wheat flour, whole grain breakfast cereals.
All foods listed above are assumed free of fats, oils, eggs and
sweeteners.

Any combination of legumes and whole grains should result in high-quality protein.

•FATIGUE FIGHTER #11-A: Ten Energy Boosters from the Sports Nutrition World

The goal of sports nutritionists is to find foods, and ways
of eating them, that enable athletes to maximize the performance of their energy mechanisms. Yet you needn't be an
athlete to benefit from sports nutrition. The following ten
tips—all researched and confirmed by leading sports nutrition
groups—can help anyone become a high energy person.

•Energy Booster #1.

Eat a generous breakfast every day followed by a moderate-sized lunch and a light dinner. Researchers have repeatedly found that people who skip breakfast, or who eat

refined carbohydrates like doughnuts and sweet rolls with coffee in place of breakfast, frequently experience chronic tiredness.

In a study of the lifestyle habits of 7,000 people in Alameda County, California, researcher James Enstrom Ph.D., found that eating breakfast daily was one of seven habits directly linked with living a long, healthy life. All of the longest-lived participants in the study ate breakfast regularly. But for men who frequently skipped breakfast, the death rate was 40 percent higher, and for women it was 28 percent higher, than for those who ate breakfast regularly.

Other studies have repeatedly found that skipping breakfast, or eating doughnuts or a Danish, not only causes low energy but reduces memory, concentration and reading skills.

Ideally, breakfast should consist of a cooked or cold whole grain cereal with fresh fruit plus half a cup or more of plain nonfat yogurt to add protein. Coffee should be avoided. Cooked cereals can be prepared the night before and kept warm in a thermos or crock pot. Should you miss breakfast, be sure to eat some kind of complex carbohydrate snack before getting to work. Otherwise, you may be drained of energy by eleven o'clock.

At all costs, avoid a light breakfast and a heavy dinner at night. And try to eat your three main meals at roughly the same time each day.

•Energy Booster #2.

Most sports nutritionists agree that no limit need be placed on the amount of complex carbohydrate foods you eat. You should endeavor to cut back only on fat and animal protein. In fact, the more fruits, vegetables, whole grains and legumes you eat, the less room there is for excess fat and protein. Provided they consist entirely of complex carbohydrates, unlimited snacks are also okay.

As far as possible, try to eat about the same amount of food each day. Avoid drastic ups and downs in quantity.

•Energy Booster #3.

The fastest way to replenish energy used in exercise is to drink a large glass of water and to eat a hi-carb snack immediately after exercising and another snack one hour later. Each snack should consist of .5 grams of complex carbohydrate for every pound you weigh. For a 150 pound person, this equals 75 grams or 300 calories. This can translate into a bowl of cereal and a banana for one snack and a bowl of vegetable soup and some whole grain crackers for the second snack.

This advice stems from studies by sports nutritionists which revealed that a hi-carb snack eaten immediately after exercising is rapidly converted into glucose and supplies 50 percent more glycogen and energy to muscles than if the same food were eaten two hours after exercise ends. Another recent study found that eating within two hours after exercising replaced glycogen three times faster than if you wait two to four hours before eating.

Sports nutritionists have concluded that the glycogen recovery rate is fastest during the first two hours after exercising. If you wait longer before eating, it takes significantly longer to recover your energy.

For this advice to be effective, however, you must drink

abundant amounts of water. Otherwise, your energy will take longer to recover.

•Energy Booster #4.

Once you begin walking, or commence any other continuous, rhythmic exercise, you will need a hi-carb snack between the second and third hours. After that, you must snack every hour to maintain glycogen levels.

For instance, a 150 pound man bicycling at 15 m.p.h. burns 500 calories per hour. Assuming the rider eats a full hi-carb meal an hour or two before beginning to ride, he could typically expect to go for 120 to 150 minutes (burning 1,000 to 1,250 calories) before needing a snack. Because women have a smaller lean muscle mass for storing glycogen, a woman would probably need a snack after riding for 105 to 130 minutes.

When exercising continually for a long period, one's carbohydrate energy resources are steadily depleted. After getting two hours or so into the exercise, a man needs to begin eating a 75 gram complex carbohydrate snack at hourly intervals. A woman should eat at slightly shorter intervals. Without regular snacks to replenish glucose and glycogen supplies, the body will turn to burning fat instead.

Even though you may not plan on walking for several hours at a stretch, this research demonstrates how even athletes can become fatigued unless refuelled by regular complex carbohydrate snacks.

For healthy, high energy snacks, consider bananas; whole grain fig bars, bagels or muffins; a baked potato, fat-free granola bars, whole grain bread spread with jam, jelly, marmalade or honey; sunflower seeds and raisins, or trail mix. Trail mix consists of seeds, peanuts, dried fruits, sliced nuts and cooked dried grains mixed together; it is available ready-mixed at outdoor and natural food stores.

•Energy Booster #5.

You can build up energy reserves for an upcoming event by loading up beforehand on complex carbohydrate foods. Sports nutritionists call it "carbohydrate loading." For several days preceding a long race, or a long all-day hike or bicycle ride, athletes eat meals composed almost entirely of complex carbohydrates. By the day of the event, this ensures that the liver and muscles are loaded with glycogen. Finally, on the morning of the event, they eat another hi-carb meal. Then, during the day, they will snack at regular intervals as described in Energy Booster #4.

Tubers and whole grains, similar to the Power Foods listed in FF#7, are most popular for carbohydrate loading. Although intended to provide energy for fairly strenuous events, carbohydrate loading can be used by anyone to boost energy reserves for an upcoming activity.

•Energy Booster #6.

Drink plenty of fluids. Since it takes copious amounts of water to digest complex carbohydrates, sports nutritionists advise drinking eight to twelve glasses of water, or other fluids, daily. Drinking less can cause one to feel tired. In fact, many sports nutritionists believe that the majority of Americans are suffering from borderline dehydration.

The color of your urine is a good indication of your fluid needs. If it is brown or dark yellow, and you are not urinating at reasonable intervals, you may well need more water. During the day, urine should be clear and should be excreted in significant amounts at regular intervals.

Caffeine, or caffeinated soft drinks, including diet varieties, may act as diuretics and contribute to dehydration. Most sports nutritionists also agree that, while sports drinks are not harmful, neither are they necessary. The same energy supplied by a sports drink can be obtained by eating a banana and drinking a glass of water.

•Energy Booster #7.

Avoid crash diets. Diets that cause excessive calorie cutting not only deplete your energy but also lead to irritability, inability to concentrate and wild mood swings. If you're trying to lose weight, cutting out fat and increasing intake of complex carbohydrates, plus a regular, daily exercise program, should take your weight gradually down to its optimal level. Then, for as long as you stay with the hi-carb diet and the exercise, your weight should remain normal.

Instead, crash diets slow metabolism, as the body tries frantically to store calories. Restrictive diets inevitably end with a binge and eventually the dieter will regain all the weight—and more—she may have lost. In reality, most women need a minimum of 1,250 to 1,500 calories per day and men 1,500 to 2,000. Consuming fewer calories may create a deficiency of key nutrients essential to the functioning of the energy mechanism.

Avoid skipping meals, especially breakfast, to lose weight. It causes you to eat more later in the day. And eating a large meal late in the evening is a guaranteed way to add weight.

•Energy Booster #8.

Eliminate the Postprandial Dip. If you're hit by an energy slump around 3:00 p.m. each afternoon, it could be due to what you ate for lunch. To stay alert through the afternoon, avoid eating a heavy lunch, especially one with any fat or fried foods or alcohol. Many nutritionists recommend starting off with some protein, preferably beans with a whole grain. Alternatively, a small helping of tuna fish or sardines is permissible. The remainder of your lunch should consist of a large vegetable salad with peas, seeds, sprouts and tofu.

Bread, pasta, potatoes, candy bars, dried fruits, sweeteners and soda drinks may also decrease alertness. To some extent, the mid-afternoon slump may be due to circadian rhythms which intensify with age. This influence can be largely offset by getting a sound night's sleep.

•Energy Booster #9.

Most people are advised to switch gradually to a diet high in complex carbohydrates. Otherwise, the sudden jump in fiber level may induce flatulence or bloating. You can minimize gas, however, by soaking all legumes for six hours or overnight and discarding the water before cooking; and by avoiding meals which contain both beans and any member of the cabbage family. Most high fiber foods also call for more chewing than those we may be used to. Despite these cautions, most people can make the transition to eating 30 or more grams of fiber daily in just a short time.

Keep salt to one pinch per meal. It has no energy value and a large intake can contribute to muscle tension and kidney damage.

•Energy Booster #10.

Several sports nutritionists report that eating six or more equal-sized mini-meals spaced out during the day may help stabilize blood sugar levels. To eat the mini-meal way, you divide your entire day's food supply into six or more equal portions and eat one mini-meal every two hours or so. For instance, you might eat one mini-meal on rising, another before leaving for work, one at the mid-morning break, one at lunch, one during the mid-afternoon break, one on arriving home and the remainder spread out during the evening. Obviously, mini-meals eaten away from home would be portable snacks, while cooked meals could be eaten at home.

Be sure that the total food consumed in the form of mini-meals does not exceed the amount of food you normally would consume in a day. Diabetics should adopt a mini-meal routine only with a physician's cooperation.

Spices such as cinnamon and turmeric not only add zest to cooking but may help the energy mechanism. A recent in vitro study by Richard A. Anderson Ph.D., of the Human Nutrition Research Center, USDA, discovered that these two spices tripled the ability of insulin to metabolize glucose. While no human studies have yet been done, it wouldn't hurt to sprinkle some cinnamon on your oatmeal and to use some turmeric when making curried rice. People who have sampled these spices report improved blood sugar control.

Also not scientifically validated yet is a discovery made some years ago by Thomas K. Cureton Jr., Ph.D., director of the Physical Fitness Institute at the University of Illinois from 1950 to 1972. While observing the effect of eating wheat germ on athletes over a 22-year period, Cureton found measurable proof that eating wheat germ lowers the pulse rate, improves stamina and endurance, and increases the rest

145

period of the heart while exercising, thus improving resistance to every type of stress. It may very well be the vitamin E in wheat germ that produces these effects.

Cureton recommended eating half a cup of fresh wheat germ per day. Fresh wheat germ is available in health food stores and should be stored in the refrigerator. Sprinkling some of this healthy, nutrient-rich food on your breakfast cereal certainly wouldn't hurt.

•FATIGUE FIGHTER #11-B: How to Stop Food Allergies from Destroying Your Energy

A hidden food allergy may be causing all or part of your chronic tiredness. In some people, certain foods may trigger the same type of reaction as do caffeine, cigarettes or alcohol. Though the effect of food is usually milder, nevertheless a specific food which we eat often and in large quantities may stimulate the adrenals to boost the blood sugar level in the same way as stronger stimulants.

Feeling fatigued a short time after eating a favorite food is frequently a strong indicator of a biochemical sensitivity to that food.

When we eat this food the immune system recognizes it as a threat and turns on some or all of the fight or flight mechanisms. This signals the adrenals to release hormones that raise the blood sugar level and send glucose surging into the muscles, priming them for emergency action.

For an hour or so we feel terrific and filled with energy. But because we repeatedly eat this same food, the adrenals soon become exhausted. In one or two hours after eating an allergenic food, our energy level plummets and we swiftly feel fatigued again. The only solution is another fix of the culprit food. Pretty soon, we develop a full-scale addiction to this food. If we don't eat it regularly, we begin to feel listless and unable to concentrate.

These discomforting feelings are actually withdrawal symptoms. And the simplest way to end them is to eat another fix of the addictive food.

Obviously, the solution is to identify this gremlin food and cease to eat it regularly. But before you can do this you must first have overcome any addiction to stronger stimulants such as caffeine, nicotine or alcohol (see Chapter 7). Once you have eliminated these toxins from your body, identifying addictive foods becomes relatively easy.

The simplest way to uncover a hidden food allergy is to answer the following questions by making a list of the relevant foods (or beverages):

1. Must you eat any particular food, such as dairy, wheat or sugar in some form at every meal to feel satisfied?

2. Must you have a certain food for breakfast before you feel able to face the day?

3. Must you eat a specific food just before bedtime in order to fall asleep?

4. Must you have any specific food at lunch or for between-meal snacks?

5. Which foods would you miss most if they were no longer available?

6. Do you experience discomfort if you are late for a meal or miss a meal containing certain foods?

7. Could you relieve this discomfort by eating these foods?

8. Do you always stock up on certain specific foods because of a compulsive fear of running out?

147

9. Does eating a certain food always seem to be followed by increased tiredness, fatigue or mental dullness?

10. Do certain foods almost invariably cause heartburn, indigestion, gas or gastrointestinal problems of any type?

Typically, the foods you have listed may well include such common food allergens as cow's milk and dairy products; red meat, chicken or pork; bacon, sausage, hot dogs or luncheon meats; chocolate; yeast; cane or beet sugar and molasses; food colorings, dyes and additives; eggs; shellfish; and soft drinks, especially caffeinated sodas.

You may also develop a biochemical sensitivity to even the healthiest complex-carbohydrate foods. Wheat, corn and soy (including TVP, textured vegetable protein) are also common allergenic foods, as are citrus, peanuts, white potatoes, bell peppers, tomatoes, garlic and some types of peas or beans.

Head your list with the food you crave most, eat most frequently and consume most of. Then list the remainder in decreasing order.

To identify which of these foods may be causing your fatigue, you simply eliminate one food at a time for a five-day period. Suppose that wheat is at the top of your list. Starting with breakfast tomorrow, you eliminate all foods containing wheat for the next five days. If during this time, you experience no symptoms of tiredness, dullness or fatigue and no craving for wheat, then wheat is probably not causing your fatigue.

On the sixth day you may reintroduce wheat back into your diet. On this same day you eliminate from your diet the second food on your list of suspected allergens. Let's assume it is red meat. For the next five days, including all of today, you totally eliminate any form of red meat from your diet.

Let's say that by the third day you feel unusually dull and listless and that you experience a strong craving for some beef, hamburger or other red meat. This would be a good indication that you are addicted to red meat and that a sensitivity to red meat may be the cause of all or part of your chronic weariness and fatigue.

If this happens, omit red meat from your diet entirely while you complete a similar five-day elimination test for each of the remaining foods on your list.

Assuming that none of these other foods showed a sensitivity, you should have reintroduced them all back into your diet. And without red meat in your diet, you should now be feeling more alive and energetic.

To confirm red meat's addictive role, you should introduce it back into your diet once more. If you again experience a reaction, you can be fairly certain that, for you, red meat is an allergenic food. So remove it once more from your diet.

This doesn't mean you must never eat red meat again. Usually it is the quantity of a food that is eaten, and the frequency, that causes it to become addictive. So after having abstained from red meat completely for, say, 15 days, you can reintroduce it on a rotation basis. That means you may eat a moderate helping of red meat once—and only once—every four days. Should red meat again trigger a reaction, it should be eliminated altogether. But most allergenic foods may be safely eaten once in each four day period.

It's important to realize that only primary foods may be tested. If you test positive to a hamburger, are you sensitive to the meat or to the wheat bun, the tomato, lettuce, mayonnaise or mustard? An addiction to pizza could mean you have a sensitivity to the cheese or to the wheat in the crust, the vegetables or the spices or seasonings. Commercial breads, and many prepared and manufactured foods, also consist of a combination of primary foods.

Obviously, if an elimination test identifies pizza, hamburger, bread or any other multiple food as an allergen, you should eliminate it and eat it only on a rotational basis. However, you can often identify the exact culprit food by separately testing each of the ingredients in a combination food.

Naturally, if you do not get a reaction to any of your suspect foods, you are probably free of any food addiction problem.

A final caution: do not attempt this technique without your doctor's approval if you have diabetes or are under a doctor's care for any nutrition-related disorder, or if you have any condition which elimination and reintroduction of a food might worsen.

CHAPTER NINE

Nutrients That Boost Energy

Gulping megadoses of vitamins and minerals is not a likely panacea for chronic tiredness. Nor do vitamins or minerals contain any energy.

Yet the body relies on a total of more than 40 vitamins, minerals and other nutrients to augment efficient functioning of the energy mechanism. Without key nutrients, neither carbohydrates nor fats could be transformed into energy nor could oxygen reach the muscles.

Among their many vital roles, both vitamins and minerals are enzyme activators. That is, they act as co-enzymes to the body's own enzymes during chemical reactions that liberate energy from food.

Vitamin and mineral supplements may be unnecessary if you eat a well-balanced variety of predominently complex carbohydrate foods. But a recent CDC survey showed that fewer than nine per cent of Americans consume the bare minimum of fruits and vegetables considered essential for adequate nutrition. Even those who eat sufficient complex carbohydrates may lose essential nutrients through overcooking. Diuretics and other prescription drugs deplete older Americans of potassium and magnesium. In fact, millions of Americans are deficient in magnesium, a mineral vital to energy production.

The constant simmering of the fight or flight response during the prolonged stresses of modern living is another widespread source of nutrient depletion. Among vitamins and minerals consumed by stress are vitamins B-1, B-5 and B-6, vitamin C, and chromium, iron, magnesium, potassium and zinc. Any deficiency of these nutrients may inhibit performance of the energy mechanism and result in fatigue.

As people age, malabsorption and poor assimilation become increasingly common, especially of the fat-soluble vitamins A, D, E and K.

Meanwhile, the RDA listed for each nutrient is the bare minimum needed to sustain life and to prevent diseases like pellagra and scurvy. Scores of studies have shown that, due to poor diet and poor absorption, millions of men and women do not even get the RDAs of many nutrients. And to prevent chronic tiredness, many individuals may need more than basic RDA levels.

DEFICIENCIES THAT CAUSE FATIGUE

A deficiency of folic acid, or vitamin C, or of iron, magnesium, potassium or zinc may readily lead to chronic tiredness. Studies show that millions of Americans have a mild deficiency of iron or magnesium or both, especially teenagers, the elderly, the poor, people under stress, dieters, those taking medications and people who smoke or consume alcohol.

For instance, in a recent test at a university medical center, a group of people with chronic fatigue reported that their energy level had increased 50 percent after taking a supplement of magnesium- and potassium-aspartate for three months.

One problem is that while blood levels of vitamins and minerals can be measured, a mild deficiency is difficult to detect. Yet due to poor absorption, many older Americans have a subtle deficiency of nutrients, especially vitamin B-12. For example, a recent study by Robert H. Allen, M.D., director of hematology at the University of Colorado Health Sciences Center, found that conventional blood tests failed to show any blood abnormalities in 141 out of 323 people diagnosed with a deficiency of vitamin B-12. A similar study by Ralph Carmel, Ph.D., at the University of Southern California, also revealed that out of 70 people with vitamin B-12 deficiency, 23 showed no abnormality in routine blood tests. The authors concluded that a subtle deficiency of vitamin B-12 may be much more common than most doctors assume.

All too many doctors may also assume that a low B-12 reading may be merely a borderline case or a lab error. Unless anemia or other blood abnormalities show up on the same test, some doctors may ignore a subtly low B-12 level. Undoubtedly the same could be said for other key nutrients. Hence even routine blood tests may not always reveal deficiencies that could contribute to fatigue.

153

A DEFICIENCY THAT SHOWS UP ONLY
DURING EXERCISE

Certain deficiencies may also show up only after exercising. For instance, Erik Van Der Beek, a nutrition and sports medicine authority at the Toxicology and Human Nutrition Institute in Zeist, Netherlands, created a mild vitamin deficiency in 23 men by cutting back their intake of vitamins B-1, B-2, B-6 and C by one-third of the U.S. RDA levels for eight weeks. While resting or during routine activity, the men showed no vitamin deficiency. But when they exerted themselves during exercise, Van Der Beek and his colleagues discovered an average decrease of ten percent in aerobic capacity and a 20 percent decrease in endurance.

Although the vitamin deficiency was mild, even subtle, it was sufficient to cause a significant drop in the efficiency of the men's energy mechanisms. Actually, these water-soluble vitamins are essential to the body's ability to draw on fat to supplement glucose as a muscle fuel during prolonged exercise. Even a slight deficiency significantly impaired the body's endurance and aerobic capacity.

WATER-SOLUBLE VITAMINS MUST BE
REPLACED DAILY

Water soluble vitamins, such as the B-complex and C, are most likely to be deficient in people with chronic tiredness. That's because these nutrients cannot be stored in the body and must be replaced each day. These same vitamins are also those used up most rapidly while under stress.

The necessity of B-1, or thiamine, was demonstrated recently during a study of 80 women in Ireland with moderate thiamine deficiency by the department of nutrition at the University of California, Davis. When the women were given a daily thiamine supplement, levels of fatigue and insomnia diminished and appetite and general well-being significantly improved.

Vitamin B-6 is equally essential for increasing stamina and preventing fatigue. In the *Journal of Sports Medicine and Physical Fitness* (June 1981), John H. Richardson, M.D., a biology professor at Old Dominion University in Norfolk, Va., reported on a B-6 study made on animals. Two groups of 20 rats each were fed the same rat diet for 30 days and given workouts on an exercise wheel. One group also received oral B-6 supplementation.

At the end of the 30-day period, each group was tested for stamina and time of fatigue. The tests revealed that muscle contraction time for the B-6 supplemented rats was significantly better than for the controls. Although it remains to be tested on humans, indications are that B-6 supplementation may well increase stamina.

Obviously, a higher intake of vitamins and minerals may maximize the body's energy mechanism potential. Without very adequate levels of B-5, inositol and magnesium, for instance, ATP production drops and a person experiences extreme fatigue.

ENERGY-BOOSTING SUPPLEMENTS

For most people, a hi-carb diet could supply all of the body's energy nutrients. But for those who do not eat ideally, or who may have an absorption problem, supplements may help.

In most cases, a high-potency vitamin-mineral supplement will do the job. Because some cheaper brands tend to over-emphasize the B-complex at the expense of minerals, we suggest checking to see that your supplement is well-balanced. For superior absorption we also recommend taking 100 mg twice a day rather than 200 mg once a day. And do take your supplements with meals. The food sets off enzyme reactions that improve absorption and assimilation of nutritional supplements.

By the same token, we see no reason to take megadoses of any vitamin or mineral. In fact, large amounts of vitamins A, D or K may worsen fatigue. Also, anyone under medical supervision, or who has any type of disease or dysfunction, should have medical approval before taking nutritional supplements.

The following review is intended to orient you to the role played by each key nutrient in the human energy process, and to help you identify a possible deficiency. Helpful comments on food sources and supplements are included.

Key Nutrients For Energy Production

Vitamin A.

RDA: 4,800 to 6,000 I.U. A key nutrient in preventing fatigue, vitamin A helps prevent anemia and maintains the integrity of red blood cells that carry oxygen to the muscles. The best vegetable source (also known as beta-carotene) is found in dark green and yellow-orange fruits and vegetables.

It is possible to overdose on supplements, especially fish oil. Excess beta-carotene, on the other hand, is easily excreted.

Vitamin B Complex.

All B vitamins are water-soluble and easily destroyed by heat, light or cooking. A deficiency can swiftly lower one's energy level. They are also synergistic, meaning that they are more effective when the entire complex is consumed together in equal proportions. Taking a large amount of a single B vitamin might cause a deficiency of others. Various B vitamins are closely associated with each stage of the energy mechanism and are also essential to proper functioning of the liver and the adrenal glands. A teaspoon of brewer's yeast twice daily mixed with food should provide an adequate supply of most B vitamins (as well as chromium and selenium).

Vitamin B-1, Thiamine.

RDA: women 1.1 mg., men 1.5 mg. B-1 is easily depleted by eating refined carbohydrates or drinking alcohol. Teenagers and pregnant women often have a deficiency. In older people, even a marginal deficiency can lead to fatigue, depression, irritability and insomnia. B-1 is essential for conversion of carbohydrates into glucose and glycogen. Good sources are whole grains, especially brown rice; legumes, nuts, wheat germ, plain nonfat yogurt and milk, pineapple and carrots. Fish, poultry and meats are second choice sources.

Vitamin B-2, Riboflavin.

RDA: 1.3 to 1.7 mg. Essential for conversion of glucose into cellular energy, B-2 also metabolizes protein, improves thyroid function and helps assimilate iron. Good sources are apples, apricots, carrots, whole grains, plain yogurt and milk.

Vitamin B-3, Niacin.

RDA: 20 mg. B-3 acts as a co-enzyme in converting carbohydrates and fat into cellular energy. B-3 may be depleted by taking antibiotics, and a deficiency may cause chronic tiredness. In supplement form, niacin may release histamine in the body, causing a flush 15 to 20 minutes after you take it. This may be avoided by taking it in the form of niacinamide. Good food sources are leafy green vegetables, peanuts, brown rice, soybeans, wheat germ, whole wheat and sunflower seeds. It also exists in fish, poultry and dairy products.

Vitamin B-5, Pantothenic Acid.

RDA not established. One of the body's key "stress" vitamins, B-5 is easily depleted by caffeine or prolonged stress. B-5 helps prevent adrenal exhaustion and is essential for conversion of glucose into ATP. Although a true deficiency is rare, a reduced level could cause fatigue and muscular weakness and may lower resistance to stress. Good sources are legumes, whole grains, wheat germ, green leafy vegetables, cauliflower and mushrooms.

Vitamin B-6, Pyridoxine.

RDA: 2.25 mg. B-6 is vital for the release of energy from glucose or fat into muscle cells. A deficiency may be caused by caffeine, birth control pills, certain medications or exposure to radiation. Women with premenstrual syndrome often show a B-6 deficiency. Any significant deficiency may lead to chronic tiredness or anemia. As a supplement it should be taken only with other B vitamins; an excess may cause nerve damage. Good sources are whole grain products, wheat germ, avocados, bananas, cabbage, cauliflower, dried fruits, nuts and rice. It also exists in beef, eggs, poultry and dairy products.

Vitamin B-9, Folic Acid.

RDA: 400 micrograms. This fragile nutrient is easily depleted by alcohol, antibiotics, birth control pills, caffeine, overcooking, smoking, stress, chemotherapy or certain medications, and millions of Americans are believed to have a mild deficiency. Folic acid helps prevent anemia and is crucial to formation of red blood cells. Thus a pronounced deficiency can lower energy and induce depression, lethargy or insomnia. Since folic acid supplementation may affect B-12 supplementation, folic acid is best taken as part of the entire B-complex. Good sources include apricots, avocados, cantaloupes, dates, legumes, pumpkins, whole wheat products, oranges, potatoes, leafy green vegetables and plain nonfat yogurt or milk.

Vitamin B-12, Cobalamin.

RDA: 6 micrograms. Although needed only in microscopic amounts, B-12 is essential for maintaining the myelin which sheaves the nervous system. It is also vital to red blood cell formation. Thus any deficiency may lead to pernicious anemia; to symptoms of fatigue or depression; to nerve deterioration; or to memory loss or confusion. While B-12 can be depleted by alcohol, caffeine, a deficiency of B-6, or inadequate calcium intake, a severe deficiency of B-12 is

159

usually found only in older people who have an absorption problem. Since B-12 exists only in animal foods, strict vegetarians may eventually develop a deficiency. A deficiency of B-12 could have serious consequences. Fortunately, it responds well to B-12 injections and symptoms usually soon disappear. To maintain levels, fortified breakfast cereals or oral supplementation also work well in most people. Should you have gas or indigestion after taking B-12 supplements, it may indicate an absorption problem. Unfortunately, B-12 exists only in meat, fish, poultry, eggs and dairy foods. Soybean foods such as tempeh are not considered a dependable source.

Other B-vitamins such a biotin, choline, inositol or PABA (para-aminobenzoic acid) are also valuable fatigue fighters. Good sources are whole grains, especially brown rice, oatmeal or wheat germ; mushrooms, peanuts, soybeans and plain nonfat yogurt or milk.

Vitamin C, Ascorbic Acid.

RDA: 40 to 60 mg. An important nutrient and antioxidant, vitamin C plays a key role in maintaining the health of the adrenal glands and also helps the body to absorb iron. Yet it can be steadily used up by physical exercise or by prolonged stress. Vitamin C is also depleted by antibiotics, aspirin, birth control pills and smoking. A severe deficiency can result in chronic tiredness or physical weakness. Many people rely on oral supplements to increase their intake far beyond RDA levels. Simple ascorbic acid in powder form, dissolved in water or in fruit juice cut with water, is considered a cheap and dependable source. Good food sources include all berries, broccoli, cauliflower, citrus, green leafy vegetables, green peppers, potatoes, sweet potatoes, strawberries, tomatoes and turnip greens.

Vitamin D.

RDA: 400 I.U. Essential to the absorption of calcium and for functioning of the thyroid gland, vitamin D is normally supplied by the action of sunshine on the skin. Milk is also fortified with vitamin D. However, in cloudy climates or for older, house-bound people, some nutritionists suggest a supplement of 200 to 400 I.U. daily. Your physician's approval is suggested before taking supplements.

Vitamin E.

RDA: 30 I.U. Crucial to maintaining the integrity of red blood cells and to the health of the thyroid gland, Vitamin E makes an important contribution to the efficient performance of the energy mechanism. While this vitamin is also an important antioxidant, as far as energy is concerned, most people appear to have an adequate intake.

Perhaps the best way to ensure an adequate intake is to sprinkle a liberal helping of fresh wheat germ on your breakfast cereal. (See the final two paragraphs under FF #11-A, Energy Booster #10.) Wheat germ is an excellent source of vitamin E. Alternatively, you could take a daily supplement of 200 I.U. Before taking a higher amount, we suggest checking with your physician.

Calcium.

RDA: 800 to 1200 mg. Calcium is the principal nutrient that prevents muscle fatigue. A deficiency could significantly

161

decrease stamina and endurance. Calcium may be depleted by a diet high in fat and animal protein and by lack of exercise or prolonged stress. Many nutritionists recommend a supplement of 600 mg. per day; after menopause or age 50, women should take one gram. Any calcium supplement should include magnesium. Good food sources are broccoli, brussel sprouts, carrots, grapefruit, green leafy vegetables, plain nonfat yogurt or milk, or water-packed sardines or salmon (eat the bones!).

Chromium.

RDA not established. In the form of Glucose Tolerance Factor (GTF), trace amounts of chromium are essential for the release of insulin to maintain glucose levels in the blood-stream and to store glycogen. Many American diets are known to be low in chromium and deficiency is common, particularly in older persons and diabetics. Most refined car-bohydrates have been stripped of chromium. A deficiency may lead to chronic tiredness and cause erratic blood sugar levels or diabetes. Supplementation is by taking GTF chro-mium or chromium picolinate, usually 250 to 400 micro-grams daily in a multiple vitamin-mineral tablet. Good dietary sources include bananas, brewer's yeast, mushrooms, peas, potatoes and whole grains.

Copper.

RDA: 2 mg. Copper works with zinc to regulate thyroid function and with iron to form hemoglobin. Taking longer than usual to fall asleep may possibly indicate a deficiency. If you supplement, never exceed the RDA. Levels as low as 10 mg. may be toxic. The best sources are almonds, avocados, bananas, beans, dried prunes, mushrooms, tofu and walnuts.

Iron.

RDA: 10 mg. for males and postmenopausal women; 18 mg. for women of childbearing age. Generally found only in women, and easily corrected by oral supplements, iron-deficiency anemia is one of the most common causes of chronic tiredness. Without adequate dietary iron, the body is unable to produce sufficient hemoglobin to enable red blood cells to transport oxygen throughout the body. And without ample oxygen to transform glucose into ATP, muscle fatigue sets in, accompanied by anemia.

Common symptoms of iron-deficiency anemia are apathy, pallor, shortness of breath, depression, difficulty in concentrating and a constant devastating tiredness. Anemic people always feel sluggish, are barely able to perform routine tasks, and are totally exhausted by any strenuous activity. However, not all women with iron-deficiency anemia are affected equally. Some women with anemia barely feel it while others with only a mild iron deficiency experience constant fatigue.

Iron-deficiency anemia is most common among women who are pregnant, nursing or menstruating heavily. It may also affect both men and women who have undergone recent surgery or have a bleeding injury or who may have an iron deficiency. Most cases in men are due to ulcers, hemorrhoids, gastrointestinal tract bleeding or cancer. Many younger women also have borderline anemia, as do many alcoholics, people on strict diets and those who live on junk food. Millions of American women may not get the RDA for iron.

Iron-deficiency anemia should be detected by your physi-

163

cian during the obligatory medical checkup recommended in Chapter 2. A hemoglobin test can be ordered as part of a screening blood panel. The result shows the percentage of blood cells that are red, and the capacity of the blood to carry oxygen. If the test shows a decreased number of red cells with a below-average size, your doctor may diagnose iron-deficiency anemia.

Oral supplementation that combines iron with vitamin C (to aid absorption) is then prescribed and chronic tiredness begins to disappear. When all symptoms are gone, you can continue with a multiple vitamin-mineral capsule containing vitamin C and 18 mg. of iron. If you supplement on your own, you should never exceed 18 mg. of iron per day.

Aside from red meat and liver (which should be minimized because of their high fat content) food sources of dietary iron are chicken, fish, shellfish and eggs. Dairy products are low in iron. Many vegetables and fruits also contain iron but may be difficult to absorb without a boost from vitamin C.

There are two forms of dietary iron:

• *Heme,* the type that forms hemoglobin, exists only in animal foods, and 10 to 30 percent can be absorbed.

• *Nonheme* iron exists in plants, but only two to ten percent of the iron in plant foods can normally be absorbed by humans. Absorption of iron from plant foods can be enhanced however, when they are eaten at the same meal with meat, chicken or fish.

Among plant foods richest in iron are dried peas and beans, dried peaches and other dried fruits, green leafy vegetables, and nuts. Blackstrap molasses also has a high iron content.

To liberate more nonheme iron from plant foods, eat them

together with foods high in vitamin C, or take a vitamin C supplement immediately before eating. You can boost iron intake at breakfast, for example, by sipping a glass of orange juice along with your complex carbohydrate meal. Or cook your beans with tomatoes or bell peppers.

Since bran may bind with nonheme iron, go lightly on extra bran at breakfast if you're trying to absorb iron. Also, since calcium may bind with iron, avoid taking calcium and iron supplements together. And if you're trying to absorb iron from fortified foods, make sure that they also contain vitamin C and that the iron is either ferrous sulphate or elemental iron, both of which will be better absorbed than other types of nonheme iron.

Yet another way to absorb iron from food is to cook acidic foods (like spaghetti sauce) in cast-iron pots and pans. The iron is nonheme but a significant amount leaches into food during 15 to 20 minutes of simmering.

In view of a recent study in Finland which linked above-average blood levels of iron with increased risk for heart disease, cancer and diabetes, we advise caution in taking supplementary iron unless prescribed by your doctor. If you suspect anemia, you should have your condition diagnosed by a physician and limit iron supplementation to amounts specified by your doctor.

Magnesium.

RDA: females, 300 mg.; males, 350 mg. Magnesium sparks more chemical reactions than any other mineral and a deficiency may result in depression, heart irregularities, angina or hypertension. Magnesium is an activator of the ATP enzyme system and it plays a vital role in maintaining electrolyte balance and in transmission of nerve impulses to activate movement. A mild deficiency is enough to cause chronic tiredness. And almost every victim of CFS shows a magnesium deficiency.

In fact, preliminary findings show that CFS patients with magnesium deficiency may experience significant improvement when given injections of magnesium sulfate. In one study authored by M. J. Campbell Ph.D., of the University of Southampton General Hospital, Southampton, England, 32 CFS sufferers with low magnesium levels were divided into two groups. One group of 15 was given an intramuscular injection of magnesium sulfate each week for six weeks while the other group of 17 received a placebo. After six weeks, 12 of the group given magnesium sulfate showed a significant improvement in energy level. They also reported less pain and sounder sleep. All improvements coincided with an increased blood level of magnesium. Meanwhile, in the placebo group, only three reported any improvement. The study was reported in *Lancet*, 1991: 337; pp 757-760.

While these results appear promising, they remain preliminary. The researchers also cautioned that it is doubtful if oral supplements would have had as much effect. Nonetheless, the study clearly indicates the possibility of a powerful link between magnesium and fatigue. This seems hardly surprising when you consider that millions of Americans have been found deficient in magnesium. Magnesium depletion is common in pregnant women and older people and in those who consume alcohol, diuretics, certain medications and a high fat diet. Stress, which raises free fatty acid levels in the bloodstream, also reduced magnesium levels. Cooking can also wash magnesium out of foods. A mild deficiency does not always show up in a magnesium blood test.

See a physician if you believe you may have moderate-to-severe magnesium deficiency. If you have a kidney problem, see a physician before taking any magnesium supplement. Otherwise, if you believe you need a magnesium supplement, many nutritionists suggest taking 400 mg. per day. A larger amount may cause diarrhea.

Good food sources include whole grains, especially brown rice and oatmeal; dark green leafy vegetables; and alfalfa, apples, legumes, peanuts, nuts and seeds.

Manganese.

RDA not established. By acting as a catalyst to assist insulin in maintaining blood sugar levels, manganese helps the body release energy in response to a feeling of tiredness. As a trace mineral, 15 mg. daily is considered ample. Good food sources include fruits, vegetables, legumes, whole grains and nuts.

Potassium.

RDA: 2,000 to 2,500 mg. Studies by sports nutritionists reveal that as many as 60 percent of American men and 40 percent of women have a potassium deficiency that results in muscle weakness. Even athletes may experience a temporary potassium deficiency. If the mineral is not replaced, they experience chronic tiredness. Thus any potassium deficiency may cause chronic fatigue and muscle weakness. The body's potassium level is easily depleted by alcohol, aspirin, diuretics, steroids or stress and by a diet high in refined carbohydrates. If your doctor prescribes diuretics, ask for one that does not waste potassium. Since complex carbohydrates are rich in potassium, supplementation is rarely needed. Good

167

food sources include almost any fruit or vegetable, especially green leafy vegetables, whole grains, dried fruits, apricots, bananas, oranges, peaches, peanuts, potatoes, sunflower seeds plus plain yogurt or milk.

Selenium.

RDA: females 55 micrograms; males 70 micrograms. A study at University College, Swansea, Wales recently confirmed that a moderate deficiency of selenium can cause tiredness, depression and anxiety. When a test group was fed a diet low in selenium for an extended period, many participants displayed symptoms of fatigue, depression and anxiety. They were then given a selenium supplement of 100 micrograms per day. After a week, the group reported that their energy had normalized while their depression and anxiety had diminished. Today, many people take supplemental selenium for its antioxidant properties. But a deficiency is possible in people who avoid complex carbohydrate foods. Good food sources are broccoli, garlic, tomatoes and wheat germ, provided they are grown in selenium-rich soil.

Zinc.

RDA: 15mg. Although a trace mineral, adequate supplies of zinc are required to regulate thyroid function, to produce insulin, to transform glucose into glycogen and for muscle contraction—all essential stages in the energy mechanism. Yet millions of older Americans are believed to be zinc-deficient, especially diabetics and those who consume alcohol. Depletion may also be caused by birth control pills or by stress. A severe deficiency can lead to chronic tiredness. Good food sources include brewer's yeast, green leafy vegetables, mushrooms, onions, soybeans, sunflower seeds and wheat germ.

Coenzyme Q-10.

RDA not established. The role of this vital substance in transforming glucose into ATP is reviewed in Chapter 4 under the heading "High-Energy Duo: ATP and Coenzyme Q-10." While oral supplements of this key nutrient are available in health food stores, adequate supplies are generally available by eating bran, cereals, soybeans, nuts and dark green leafy vegetables.

•FATIGUE FIGHTER#12: Prevent Fatigue by Eating These Nutrient-Rich Foods Regularly

You can help prevent fatigue due to nutrient deficiency by making the following foods a regular part of your diet. Each of these foods is rich in one or more of the nutrients just reviewed and only two are not complex carbohydrates. If all this sounds like a lot of plant foods, remember that U.S. government guidelines recommend that we eat 2 to 4 servings of fruit each day, 3 to 5 servings of vegetables and 6 to 11 servings of whole grain foods.

•*Fruits:* apples, apricots, avocados, bananas, cantaloupe, citrus—especially oranges and grapefruit, dried fruits, dried prunes, peaches, pineapple, strawberries and yellow-orange fruits.

•*Legumes:* all beans including soybeans, chick peas, kidney beans, lentils, peas, and peanuts.

•*Nuts, Seeds:* almonds, sunflower seeds, walnuts.

•*Vegetables:* broccoli, brussels sprouts, cabbage, carrots, cauliflower, garlic, dark green leafy vegetables, bell peppers, mushrooms, onions, potatoes, pumpkins, sweet potatoes and yams, tomatoes, turnip greens and yellow-orange vegetables.

•*Whole Grains:* bran, brown rice, oatmeal, wheat germ; all breads made from whole wheat, whole grain, sprouted wheat or sprouted grain flours that contain no refined carbohydrate, fat, eggs or sweeteners (caution—most supermarket breads do not meet these requirements).

•*Others:* brewer's yeast; plain nonfat yogurt or milk.

CHAPTER TEN

Don't Let Poor Sleep Steal Your Energy

I f you need an alarm to wake up, if you are difficult to rouse, if you must sleep late on weekend mornings, if you experience daytime drowsiness, if you don't feel rested and alert on awakening—then you are probably sleep-deprived.

There is a genuine epidemic of sleep deprivation among fast-track men and women, millions of whom sleep only four to six hours each weekday night. They then try to catch up on their sleep on weekends. These people's lives are overwhelmed by schedules and demands. Yet they refuse to go to bed until everything is finished.

Poor or inadequate sleep results in symptoms that are identical to those of chronic tiredness. People who deprive them-

171

selves of sleep night after night create a sleep deficit that inhibits their energy production and leaves them feeling listless, irritable and fatigued.

A dozen recent studies have demonstrated that a person's energy level and performance suffer if they fail to get a good night's sleep. A sleep-impaired person invariably experiences loss of mental acuity accompanied by negative moods, diminished memory and reaction time, and reduced ability to make sound judgments and decisions. Chronic lack of sleep can lower a person's immunity to colds, infections and cancer and can reduce his ability to metabolize alcohol. Millions of Americans are so constantly starved for sleep that their job performance suffers. And each year, tens of thousands fall asleep at the wheel.

MOST AMERICANS NEED MORE SLEEP

Based on several recent studies, researchers have concluded that most Americans sleep 60 to 90 minutes less than they need. In seven days, they lose a full night's sleep.

For example, a recent study at Henry Ford Hospital's Sleep Disorder Research Center, Detroit, found that participants who slept an extra hour each night boosted their alertness by an average of 25 percent. In another test, students who slept 60 to 90 minutes longer each night, improved their scores in psychological tests by a similar amount.

Based on these and similar studies, sleep experts have concluded that people who get a full night's sleep enjoy better health, increased drive, productivity and creativity, more upbeat moods and greater physical energy. Even exercising and eating healthfully cannot compensate for inadequate sleep.

172

By contrast, millions of Americans who deprive themselves of sleep wake up groggy and exhausted. Over a four to six day period of sleep deprivation, daytime alertness can fall by 50 percent. Sleeping late on weekends upsets our circadian rhythm and it may not be enough to recuperate fully.

GIVE YOURSELF MORE DOWN TIME

Modern sleep studies show that most adults need eight and a half to nine hours sleep for optimal functioning, but the average adult sleeps only seven and a half hours each night. The same research has revealed that most Americans are sleeping less than people did 50 or 100 years ago and that the sleep robbers are electric light and TV, especially late-night TV. Today, we assume it's OK to sleep only six and one half hours a night when we really need eight or nine hours of sleep to feel completely vigorous and energetic.

Not only are electricity and TV stealing our sleep but so are economic pressures to work overtime or moonlight, and social pressures from friends, family and the complexities of modern life. For most people, cutting back on sleep is the only way to obtain more free time. Moreover, virtually everyone who does shift work or who works during the late evening or night hours suffers a net loss of sleep.

Clearly, sleep deprivation is a major contributing factor to chronic tiredness. Thus far, we've discussed the effects of sleep deprivation created by people who deliberately curtail their time in bed. These people sleep soundly. They simply fail to sleep for sufficient hours.

However, sleep deprivation can also be caused by insomnia. According to the National Sleep Foundation, approximately 35 percent of all adults experience difficulty in falling asleep and in maintaining sound sleep. These people spend enough hours in bed but they lie fitfully and restlessly awake instead of being asleep. The net result is also sleep deprivation.

The following action steps attempt to provide answers and solutions to both causes of sleep deprivation. FF #16-A tells how to wake up filled with energy and enthusiasm and ready to enjoy every moment of the coming day.

•FATIGUE FIGHTER #13: How to Tell If You Are Sleep Deprived

Even when quite severe, it is difficult to medically diagnose a clear physiological sleep deficit. Doctors generally rely on their patients to complain about feeling constantly groggy and tired. But according to the National Sleep Foundation, when chronic sleep deficit is allowed to continue for an extended period, a person tends to forget what it is like to be fully awake. The Foundation reports that millions of Americans live their lives in such an unrelenting fog of sleeplessness and fatigue that they become unaware of the deterioration in their daytime alertness.

Thus if you have accumulated a sleep debt over an extended period, it may be difficult to tell whether you are actually sleep deprived and how much sleep you really need.

A good way to tell is to keep notes for a two-week period. If you wake up feeling refreshed and energetic each morning, and you concentrate and perform well throughout the day, you are probably sleeping close to the optimal number of hours you require.

But if you need an alarm to wake up and are hard to rouse, and if you become drowsy while performing undemanding and repetitive sedentary tasks, you may need 30 to 60 minutes more sleep each night. If you must sleep late on weekend mornings, this strengthens the case for sleep deprivation.

Also, anything that affects your daytime alertness, including irritability, impaired work performance, poor mental acuity, mild depression, diminished memory and reaction time, and reduced ability to make sound judgments and decisions, is a good indication of insufficient sleep.

Another self-test is to lie down in mid-morning in a darkened room. If you fall asleep within five minutes, you may well need more sleep. Alternatively, if you wake up without an alarm, feeling rested and refreshed, and if you don't feel tired until bedtime, you are probably getting sufficient sleep.

If you believe you need more sleep, do this. Get up at the same time every morning. Do NOT sleep in on weekends. Instead, go to bed earlier on weekends. Also go to bed 30 to 60 or even 90 minutes earlier each weekday night.

If this sounds impractical, you may have to rethink your priorities. Most people spend an average of two and a half hours or more watching TV each evening. Shows that foster genuine inspiration, or that get you laughing, are worthwhile. But those that feature violence, or that get your adrenalin running, continue to sap your energy even while you're asleep.

Providing sufficient time for sleep is a personal problem that each of us must solve for ourselves. But anyone who is too busy to get a full night's sleep may be endangering not only his health but the quality of his work as well.

175

Chapter 12 provides many suggestions for creating a more relaxed lifestyle with more time to enjoy living and sleeping.

•FATIGUE FIGHTER #14: Overcoming Insomnia with Stimulus Control Behavior Therapy

Developed some years ago by psychologist Richard R. Bootzin, Stimulus Control Behavior Therapy beats insomnia by allowing you to remain in bed only while asleep. Since you may miss a few hours sleep during the first two or three days, it's best to begin on a Friday night.

These are the rules.

•*STEP 1.* Go to bed only when you feel tired and ready to fall asleep. Your bedtime is never fixed but when you feel drowsy and tired, you must go to bed.

•*STEP 2.* Use your bed only for sleeping or sex. Never use the telephone or watch TV or listen to radio or read or eat or do any other activity while in bed.

•*STEP 3.* Keep a clock with a lighted dial beside your bed. If you are still awake ten minutes after going to bed, get up. Go to another room and do something monotonous or routine that is neither enjoyable nor rewarding. Activities that tire the eyes such as paying bills, writing letters, reading a boring book, sewing, darning, knitting, watering plants or any kind of non-stimulating activity will do. Avoid anything strenuous or anything pleasant like eating, drinking, smoking, watching TV or reading a novel. If you like, you can try FF #17: Defuse Tension with Deep Muscle Relaxation.

176

•*STEP 4.* When you feel sleepy, return to your bed. You must associate your bed with feeling sleepy.

•*STEP 5.* If you fail to fall asleep within ten minutes, get up once more and repeat Steps 3 and 4. Keep repeating them until you fall asleep.

•*STEP 6.* If you wake up during the night and do not fall asleep within ten minutes, get up and repeat Steps 3 and 4. Keep repeating them until you fall asleep once more.

•*STEP 7.* Get up at the same time each morning every day of the week. Regardless of how poorly you may have slept, set the alarm and get up. The success of this plan hinges on your always getting up at the same rigidly fixed time. (Getting up earlier on occasion to go fishing is OK but compensate by going to sleep earlier.) Never sleep later than your fixed wake-up time. For the first few days you may feel tired but you should be okay by midday. After a few days, you should find yourself feeling drowsy and ready for bed about the same time each evening.

•*STEP 8.* Eliminate all daytime napping. Consolidate all your sleep into a single night-time pattern. And never fall asleep in front of the TV after dinner. Your night's sleep will inevitably be interrupted.

•FATIGUE FIGHTER #15: Twelve Recipes for Sound Sleep

1. Never exercise late in the evening.
2. Never consume alcohol after 7 p.m. nor caffeine after 5 p.m. Avoid using wine as a sedative at bedtime.

177

3. Before turning in, do something relaxing such as listening to restful music, reading a relaxing book, or practicing FF # 17: Defuse Tension with Deep Muscle Relaxation. Avoid reading the newspaper or weekly news magazines. They often contain sleep-disturbing material. It's also best to avoid watching TV after 9 p.m.

4. Make sure your room temperature is comfortable.

5. Avoid going to bed hungry. Sip some warm skim or nonfat milk or eat a complex carbohydrate snack with some plain, nonfat yogurt. If you wake up hungry during the night, eat a snack consisting of a slice of pineapple with a liberal helping of plain, nonfat yogurt and half an avocado. Alternatively, munch a handful of sunflower seeds and raisins.

6. Avoid a large meal late at night.

7. You can melt away tension by soaking for about 20 minutes in a hot tub bath immediately before bedtime—a natural sedative that leaves you feeling warm and relaxed.

8. Herb teas such as chamomile have a calming effect that helps induce sleep when sipped at bedtime. Other teas with natural sedative effects include catnip, hops, lemon verbena, mint, passion flower, primrose and wild thyme. Brew the tea moderately strong, stir in a teaspoon of honey and sip shortly before bedtime.

9. Go to bed when you feel tired.

10. Get up at the same time every day and never sleep later. If you're still sleepy next morning, go to bed earlier.

11. To sleep soundly and deeply throughout the night a body should be naturally tired by physical activity. So be sure to take a brisk daily walk (see FF# 3, 4 and 4-A).

12. Failure to actively use the mind by creative thinking is another major cause of insomnia. Passively watching TV

or spectator sports provides zero mental stimulation or activity. To sleep well, use and tire your mind by enrolling in a language class or by learning to play a musical instrument or by playing chess or bridge or solving logic puzzles or by doing anything at all that challenges your thinking capabilities.

•FATIGUE FIGHTER #16: Beat Sleeplessness With Paradoxical Intent

A frequent cause of sleeplessness is worrying about being unable to sleep. The more we worry about being unable to fall asleep, the less we sleep, and the more we worry.

Several sleep disorder centers report great success in beating this type of insomnia by using a technique known as *paradoxical intent*. It's based on the fact that the more we try to fall asleep, the longer we find ourselves remaining awake.

With *paradoxical intent,* you do just the opposite. You try your hardest to stay awake. The result: you usually fall asleep within a few minutes.

Studies of people using *paradoxical intent,* made at Temple University and other sleep disorder centers, have shown that the time taken to fall asleep drops dramatically. One man who usually took 57 minutes to get to sleep fell asleep in six minutes, while a woman with a sleep latency of 90 minutes was able to repeatedly fall asleep in five and a half minutes.

To use this technique, go to bed at your usual time, then attempt to remain awake by concentrating on your thoughts. Do your best to stay awake. Somehow, the effort of remaining awake tires the mind. Thus the best way to fall asleep is to try as hard as possible not to.

•FATIGUE FIGHTER #16-A: Bounce Out of Bed Each Morning Filled with Energy and Zest

With or without chronic fatigue, getting up and getting going in the morning is a formidable task for most people. But it doesn't have to be. By utilizing some of the techniques of behavioral medicine and cognitive positivism, even a person with chronic tiredness can learn to bound out of bed filled with energy and zest and impatient to begin another exciting, rewarding day.

As you may recall from Chapter 5, behavorial psychology changes the way we feel by changing the way we act. And as Chapter 11 explains, cognitive positivism can change the way you feel by changing the way you believe and think. This present action-step uses both approaches to change the way you feel about getting up and facing the day.

So never mind if you don't feel like bounding out of bed. Just do it! The very act will change the way you feel about yourself. Within seconds, you'll experience powerful feedback that will put you in full charge of your life, your energy and your drive and ambition.

Likewise, by letting go of cynical or negative beliefs, and replacing them with positive thoughts and expectations, cognitive positivism will jump-start the body by releasing a flood of excitation hormones called catecholamines.

During sleep, body temperature drops by about one degree, blood pressure falls, joints and muscles stiffen, and blood pools in the extremities. In most adults, for these physiological conditions to emerge from their sleep state, and to change back to their waking state, often takes 30 half-awake minutes and a strong cup of coffee.

Yet catecholamines can do the same job in sixty seconds—and without the caffeine. These adrenal hormones swiftly arouse the body by constricting the arteries and raising blood pressure and body temperature, and they warm up stiff joints and muscles and get venous blood flowing from the extremities. All this also primes the brain for a new day. Within two minutes of waking you can be as wide-awake and alert as most people are after being awake for half an hour.

However, to bound out of bed like a high-energy person usually requires a few minutes of preparation the night before. First, think of something you can look forward to enjoying the next day. Second, think of a goal you can look forward to accomplishing the next day. Third, think of something positive to fill your mind with immediately upon awakening.

People bound out of bed because of all the exciting things they have to look forward to during the day. The thoughts we think immediately on awakening influence our mood and outlook for the rest of the day. Thus it's important to have at least one goal, one enjoyable thing and something positive to look forward to. Waking up with pessimistic or cynical thoughts turns off the catecholamines and drains our energy.

Before turning in, place a banana on the kitchen counter and a small glass of fruit juice in the refrigerator. And, if you can, arrange to wake up to a rousing Sousa march or a lively polka.

Always get up at the same time every morning and go

to bed early enough to get a full night's sleep. Even this powerful action-step won't work as well if you are sleep-deprived. Set your alarm at least 12 minutes earlier than usual to allow sufficient time to go through the entire wake-up routine.

Mobilize Your Energy with This Wake-Up Routine

Immediately upon awakening, begin the day by filling your mind with positive thoughts and images. Look forward to having lunch with someone you enjoy or to an upcoming vacation or to a pleasant evening walk.

Then, while still under the covers, wiggle your fingers and toes and move and rotate your wrists and ankles. Stretch your face and jaw and yawn and stick out your tongue. Then close your jaw and frown. Look up, look down and swing the eyes from side to side half a dozen times. Lie back in bed and stretch out to your full length with arms overhead and arch your back.

Roll out of bed, open the curtains and—assuming it's day-light—stand before the window. Fling your arms apart and greet the day. Tell yourself, "It's great to be alive. I feel wonderful. I shall enjoy every moment of this day."

Then walk out to the kitchen and eat your banana while sipping the fruit juice. If possible, go outdoors. Ideally, weather permitting, you might walk barefooted on the grass, establishing a one-ness with nature and Mother Earth. While there, tell yourself that you will succeed at the test or the interview or the sales meeting and that you are completely ready and prepared to handle all the day's challenges.

Next, go to the bathroom and take a hot shower. Let

the water run over the back of your neck and shoulders. Because it stimulates circulation, a warm-to-hot shower is a better wake-up tonic than a cold one. Then get your skin tingling by giving yourself a brisk rub-down with a stiff towel.

Back in your bedroom, face the open window and briskly perform these limbering-up exercises. If you like, you can do them outdoors. Sunshine has a powerfully beneficial ef-·fect on the bodymind, perking up your aliveness and preparing you to enjoy every moment of the day. All the exercises are done while standing erect.

1. Raise up and down on tiptoe a dozen times to help get any remaining pooled blood up the back of your legs.

2. With legs apart and hips stationary, rotate head and shoulders all the way to the right, looking around to the right and behind you as far as possible. Repeat to the left. Swing around a dozen times from far right to far left.

3. Roll and rotate the neck in all directions.

4. Keeping the arms straight, swing them overhead, sideways, forwards and backwards a dozen times in each direction.

5. Bend forward and touch the toes six times.

6. With hands on hips, and legs straight and apart, bend the trunk sideways as far as you can six times each way.

7. Raise each knee six times as high as you can.

Each exercise can be done at a brisk pace and all should be completed within three minutes.

Finally, take five deep breaths. Inhale through the nose to the slow count of four, filling both abdomen and upper chest. Hold to the count of four. And exhale to the count of seven.

While breathing, tell yourself it's going to be a wonderful

183

day and that good things are going to happen to you throughout the day.

After this, we guarantee you won't need any coffee to wake up. But if breakfast is apt to be a rush, prepare it the night before (as described in Chapter 8 under FF# 11-A, Energy Booster #1).

CHAPTER ELEVEN

How To Tame Energy-Robbing Stress

Today, there is wide acceptance among health professionals that unresolved and unrelieved emotional stress is the underlying cause of most chronic tiredness. For millions of urban Americans, life in this pressure-cooker society exacts so much stress that it drains their energy and leaves them exhausted.

What is stress?

And why do some people seem to thrive on it and to be filled with energy, while others become anxious, depressed and chronically fatigued? More important, is it possible for someone with chronic tiredness to beat stress and to become a high-energy person?

The good news is that we *can* beat energy-robbing stress

without resorting to drugs, stimulants or expensive medical treatment. Working in stress management clinics and university medical centers, researchers have developed a variety of tools for overcoming the destructive effects of chronic stress. The three Fatigue Fighter techniques in this chapter describe how to use these discoveries to cope with, and to permanently end, the stress in your life. In the process, they can also end all psychologically-induced chronic tiredness.

The way in which emotional stress is transformed into chronic fatigue is described in detail in Chapter 4. However, before you begin using the stress management techniques in this chapter, you need to know more about the psychological origins of stress.

STRESS DEFINED

Stress is the way we feel when we are faced with a life event or lifestyle change which we *believe* threatens our security, prestige, comfort or pleasure.

Note that it's not the life event or the lifestyle change itself that creates stress. Stress is not caused by something outside us. Stress occurs inside the mind. And we create stress when we perceive the world through a filter of negative beliefs and values.

Alternatively, when we perceive life through a filter of positive beliefs and values, we seldom experience stress.

For example, both Smith and Jones work on the production line at a local plant. Both are abruptly laid off when the plant is suddenly forced to close.

Smith perceives his unemployment as a catastrophe. He sees no alternative source of employment and believes he will lose his home, furniture and car. Soon, Smith exhibits such common stress symptoms as tight shoulders and muscle tension, sweaty palms, anxiety and depression, and a growing weariness and fatigue.

Jones, on the other hand, perceives his unemployment as a welcome release from a boring, tedious job and as a wonderful opportunity to train for a new and rewarding career in electronics. Jones feels buoyant and invigorated and bounces out of bed each morning fairly bursting with energy.

Both men faced exactly the same potentially stressful life event. It wasn't the event itself, the unemployment, that was stressful. It was the way in which Smith perceived it that created his stress. The stress occurred *inside* Smith's mind. And he created it all by perceiving the world through a filter of negative and inappropriate beliefs. Soon, the stress that Smith created in his mind turned on stress mechanisms that led to chronic tiredness.

Perceiving exactly the same life event through a filter of positive beliefs, Jones achieved exactly the opposite result. He felt great, relaxed and charged with vitality.

POSITIVE THOUGHTS CHASE AWAY STRESS

A basic principle of modern psychology is that our beliefs mold our thoughts; and our thoughts mold our feelings or emotions.

In other words, the way we feel depends on the thoughts we were recently thinking. Or, as psychologists put it: every feeling arises from the context of a previous thought. If you doubt this, you can easily demonstrate that your own feelings are a mirror of your thoughts.

Place a gloomy, negative thought in your mind, and hold it there, and you will soon begin to feel melancholy.

Place a thought about loss in your mind, and hold it there, and you will soon feel anxious.

Place a positive, cheerful, happy thought in your mind, and hold it there, and you will quickly begin to feel cheerful and optimistic.

We can make ourselves feel gloomy and depressed by thinking gloomy and pessimistic thoughts. We feel the way we think and, in turn, our thoughts are molded by our values and beliefs. Every negative feeling is triggered by a negative thought that arises from holding one or more negative beliefs. Likewise, every positive feeling is preceded by a positive thought that arises from holding one or more positive beliefs.

Furthermore, negative feelings turn on stress mechanisms that keep the muscles tensed and drain energy. Conversely, positive feelings keep us calm and relaxed with energy mechanisms functioning at peak efficiency.

LOVE VERSUS FEAR

Another important principle of modern psychology is that only two root emotions exist: love and fear.

• Fear-based emotions are all negative and include anger, hostility, guilt, resentment, bitterness, cynicism, frustration, envy, dissatisfaction, anxiety, depression and feeling separate from others. By the same token, all negative beliefs and values, as well as thoughts, are based on fear.

• Love-based emotions are positive and they include joy, peace, forgiveness, friendliness, generosity, compassion, contentment and experiencing a one-ness with others. Likewise, all positive beliefs and values, as well as thoughts, are based on love.

Putting it all together, this is what we get:

When you perceive the world through a filter of fear-based beliefs and values, you experience negative thoughts that turn on negative emotions that trigger stress mechanisms that drain your energy and eventually lead to chronic tiredness. This is how you create stress.

When you perceive the world through a filter of love-based beliefs and values you experience positive thoughts that turn on positive feelings that keep you calm, healthy and relaxed with your energy mechanisms charging the body with an abundance of energy. When your mind functions in this way, stress and fatigue are seldom experienced.

CHANGE THE SOFTWARE IN YOUR BIOCOMPUTER

Putting it another way, beliefs and values are the software which program the biocomputer we call the mind. When you program your biocomputer with negative beliefs, you get out negative thoughts and feelings that invariably lead to fatigue. When you program your mind with positive beliefs, you get out positive thoughts and feelings and a high level of energy.

If that sounds oversimplified, it's because we are dealing only with cause and effect. The actual bodymind mechanisms involved in the computer analogy are extremely complex.

Nonetheless, by using the computer model, researchers at

such leading medical centers as the University of Pennsylvania were able to develop several simple methodologies through which almost anyone can reprogram his or her negative beliefs and, in the process, overcome mild-to-moderate depression, anxiety, stress and psychologically-caused chronic fatigue. These methods soon proved so effective that they have virtually revolutionized the entire field of psychiatric treatment.

Since the late 1970s, most psychiatrists have gone from trying to identify problems on the couch to New Age helping techniques based on reprogramming and restructuring negative values and beliefs. These simple stress-management techniques have proved far more effective, and take far less time, than traditional psychiatric counseling.

They are so simple, in fact, that almost anyone can use them at home. By that, I mean that they are safe to use provided your doctor has given you medical clearance and is thoroughly satisfied that you do not have depression, anxiety or any other psychological or physical problem that might be exacerbated by using deep muscle relaxation, creative visualization, cognitive therapy or belief reprogramming.

HOW TO DERAIL CHRONIC FATIGUE

The stress management techniques described below are each based on behavioral medicine and each requires that you take an active role in your own recovery. Virtually all change the way you feel by changing the way you act and behave or believe.

However, they overcome stress in different ways. Through stress-coping systems like deep relaxation, you can dissipate the effects of stress after it occurs and buffer it from harming the body. Through transformational systems such as *cognitive positivism,* you can learn to prevent future stress by reprogramming your belief system so that, instead of perceiving a life event as hostile and threatening, you can see it as nonthreatening and harmless.

You can't change a life event. But you *can* change the way you react to it. By simply letting go of your negative beliefs and restructuring the mind with positive beliefs, you can triple your energy level.

The three Fatigue Fighter techniques below are presented in the order that I recommend you adopt them. FF# 17 helps you quickly release the stress-caused tension in your muscles so that you become comfortable and relaxed. As you will swiftly discover, relaxing your muscles automatically causes your mind to stop racing and to also relax.

This makes it easy for you to begin using the creative visualization methods in FF# 18. By making mental images of yourself achieving your goals, creative visulation can boost your motivation and help you succeed with any of the Fatigue Fighters in a minimum of time.

These two techniques prepare the way for FF# 18-A—restructuring your negative beliefs and values.

Naturally, if you prefer, you can begin practicing FF# 18 (creative visualization) or FF# 18-A (belief restructuring) without having practiced FF# 17 (deep relaxation) first. But I believe you will find it easier and simpler to learn and practice each technique in turn before going on to the next.

HOW TO GET STARTED

Stress management techniques must be practiced in a quiet place where you will not be disturbed. Before starting,

191

close doors and windows or use the hum of a fan or air conditioner to override any disturbing noise. Unplug the telephone. Visit the bathroom. And wipe your face and hands with a damp washrag.

Lie down on your back on a comfortable rug, or on a bed or couch, with your head supported by a pillow. Keep arms and legs straight with feet about eight inches apart and hands about eight inches from the body. Keep your eyes closed throughout.

•FATIGUE FIGHTER #17: Defuse Tension with Deep Muscle Relaxation

When you perceive a life event as threatening or hostile, you trigger stress mechanisms that energize your muscles for emergency action and that keep your shoulder, jaw and neck muscles tightly constricted. This neuromuscular tension lasts for as long as you continue to experience stress. Eventually it exhausts the adrenal glands, leading to chronic tiredness.

Since so much fatigue is caused by stress, which turns on the fight or flight response, it follows that the best way to restore energy is to stay in the opposite state, the relaxation response.

Relaxation therapy teaches that mind and body are intimately associated. When the mind is anxious or disturbed, body muscles stay tense. When body muscles are relaxed, the mind soon becomes calm and relaxed also. When the mind is relaxed, muscular tension caused by stress swiftly fades away. Relaxation therapy uses all of these principles to melt away tension.

By inducing deeper and deeper levels of relaxation, deep muscle relaxation wipes out both physical tension and the mental hyper-arousal produced by stress. Simultaneously, it releases endorphins, natural narcotics that block pain receptors in the brain and make you feel good. Deep relaxation is also the preliminary step to using creative visualization and belief restructuring.

While it will not prevent additional stress in future, it does help the body to learn to stay relaxed. Thus the effects of future stress can be lessened. Nonetheless, you will want to use deep relaxation each time that you feel tense and uptight.

Fortunately, the more you use it, the less time it takes to become completely relaxed. Many people are eventually able to achieve total mindbody relaxation in less than two minutes.

Deep muscle relaxation consists of three steps.

•STEP ONE: Learning to Identify Relaxation

During a 1986 study at the Menninger Foundation, researchers Patricia Solbach Ph.D., and Joseph Sargent M.D., discovered that many of their patients were unaware of what it felt like to be deeply relaxed. Other relaxation therapists have concluded that millions of chronically-tired men and women live in an unbroken state of emergency arousal and may not have experienced genuine relaxation in many years.

To achieve deep relaxation, you must first learn to recognize exactly what relaxation is and how it differs from tension.

So lie comfortably on a rug, bed or couch with arms extended slightly from the sides.

Raise the right arm so that the hand is about six inches off the floor. Make a fist and tense the entire lower arm and hand. Tense and squeeze as tightly as you can and hold.

Now become aware of the very uncomfortable feeling in

193

your right arm and hand as you hold it under tension. Hold the tension for only six seconds. Then release and gently lower the arm. Experience how good it feels as your right arm and hand become immediately relaxed.

Without waiting, repeat the same routine using the left arm. As you hold the left arm tensed, compare how it feels with the now-relaxed right arm. Hold your left arm tightly tensed for six seconds. Then release and gently lower it.

Never again should you have any difficulty identifying muscular tension. Many fatigued people experience such constant tension in the jaw that it aches continually and causes constant frowning.

Mentally work over your eyes, face, forehead, jaw and neck and identify tense areas. Most of us can readily identify tension around the eyes. Much of this stems from anxiety, hostility or cynicism. But it may become so habitual that it persists even after the emotions themselves have disappeared.

•STEP TWO: *Tensing the Muscles to Induce Relaxation*

Lie down in the relaxation position.

Raise the right leg so that the foot is about eight inches off the floor or bed. Tense the entire leg—that is, the muscles of the toes, foot, calf and thigh—as hard as you can. Curl and squeeze the toes tightly. Keep tensing as hard as you can while you count off approximately six seconds. Then release and lower the leg gently to the floor.

Repeat with the left leg.

Do not move any limb once it has been tensed and released.

Next, tense both buttocks as hard as you can. Hold six seconds and release.

194

In the same way, tense the abdomen muscles as if you were about to be punched in the belly. Hold six seconds and release.

Force the shoulder blades down, back and together as if trying to make the blades touch. Tense the shoulders and blades, hold six seconds and release.

Then hunch the shoulders all the way forward. Tense tightly for six seconds and release.

Raise the right arm so that the hand is eight inches off the floor. Make a fist and tense the muscles of the upper arm, forearm, hands and fingers. Tense as tightly as you can for six seconds, then release. Lower the arm gently back to the floor.

Repeat with the left arm.

Press the back of your head into the pillow and arch your neck as you lift the shoulders clear off the floor or mattress. Hold six seconds and release. Then, without raising the head off the pillow, roll it loosely from side to side a few times.

The face comes next.

Without forcing or straining your eyes, roll them upwards and look up. Raise the eyebrows as high as you can. Tense the scalp and wrinkle the forehead by squeezing it hard. Hold for six seconds and release.

Next, look down, drop the eyebrows as much as you can, and squeeze the forehead into a frown. Hold six seconds and release.

Squeeze the eyes shut, squeeze your cheeks, wrinkle your nose, press your tongue against your upper front teeth (assuming you don't wear dentures), purse your lips and clench your jaw. Tense and hold for six seconds and release.

Give a wide, deep yawn. Relax all facial muscles by breaking into a broad smile. Visualize your forehead as being very cool and picture a wave of restful calm drifting down over your face. Then flow on without pause into Step 3.

•STEP THREE: Going Deeper into Relaxation

Begin this step by taking five slow, deep breaths. With each breath, fill the abdomen as well as the upper chest. Then resume normal breathing.

Place the awareness on the soles of your feet. Repeat these phrases silently to yourself. "My feet feel relaxed. Relaxation is flowing into my feet. My feet feel deeply relaxed. Relaxation is filling my legs. My lower legs are limp and relaxed. Relaxation is flowing into my thighs. My thighs feel limp and relaxed."

You don't need to repeat these exact words. But do give yourself essentially the same suggestions. As you mentally relax each part of your body, place your awareness on that area and visualize it as limp and relaxed. For instance, you could picture your thighs filled with cotton and as limp and relaxed as a piece of old, worn-out rope.

Continue telling yourself, "My buttocks feel limp and relaxed. My buttocks feel like they're filled with cotton. My abdomen is limp and relaxed. My neck and shoulders are limp and relaxed. My hands and arms are limp and relaxed. My entire body feels as limp and relaxed as a rag doll."

If you detect the dull ache of tension anywhere in your body, mentally relax it before going on.

Place the awareness on the face as you say, "My scalp is relaxed. My forehead feels smooth and relaxed. My eyes are quiet. My face is soft and relaxed. My tongue is relaxed. My mouth is relaxed. My jaw is slack."

Watch carefully for any areas of tension in the temple, jaws, eyes or face. As you repeat the suggestions, visualize

196

the tense facial areas filled with cotton until the tension fades.

Finally, tell yourself, "My entire mind and body are deeply relaxed. I am in a state of deep relaxation."

At this stage, your breathing should have slowed and you should be taking deep, slow, relaxed breaths. You can now deepen your relaxation by using the "spring visualization."

Picture yourself in a beautiful garden facing a deep, transparent spring. So clear is the water that you can plainly see the white sandy bottom one hundred feet below.

Now, imagine yourself tossing a shiny new dime into the spring. Then, from a distance of about two feet, watch the dime as it twists and flashes and darts and rolls on its slow, silent way to the bottom. Watch the dime closely as it drifts down and down, deeper and deeper. After a minute, it comes to rest on the white sandy bottom. Here, in the depths of the spring, far from freeways and telephones, pressure and deadlines, all is completely calm, peaceful, relaxed and still.

Tell yourself again, "My mind and body are deeply relaxed. I am totally at peace and in harmony with the world. I feel only peace, joy and contentment. I am thoroughly relaxed and completely at ease."

By now, your mind should be clear and receptive and not thinking about anything in particular. Yet you should be awake and aware of everything that is going on. Let go of the past and the future. Keep your awareness in the present moment and continue to enjoy your deeply relaxed state.

WHERE TO GO FROM HERE

At this point, your body should be almost completely free of any trace of neuromuscular tension. You can continue to rest and enjoy being in the relaxation response or you can continue straight on into FF# 18 creative imagery, or FF# 18-A, belief restructuring. Both are described below.

To return to normal consciousness, remain lying down for a few moments while you open your eyes and move them around, wrinkle and unwrinkle the face, and move each muscle of the body in turn. Then sit up and move around some more. It's best to avoid getting up suddenly.

Deep relaxation can also be attained by a combination of yoga stretching postures and meditation, or by using biofeedback training. Lack of space prevents our describing these alternative techniques here. Also making deep relaxation easier to achieve are a variety of audio-cassette relaxation tapes which are widely advertised in health and New Age magazines. Whichever you use beats taking a tranquilizer.

As you become familiar with the relaxation steps, you will find yourself reaching ever-deeper levels of relaxation in less and less time. For instance, many people learn to tense and relax all of their muscles at once in a single six second period. It can be done either standing up or lying down. To practice, tense both legs at the same time. Then both arms. Then both arms and legs together. Finally, tense all the body and facial muscles that you can. If you do it standing up, lie down immediately afterwards.

Because muscle tensing calls for a brief but strenuous physical effort, anyone suffering from any form of chronic disease, or who is under medical treatment, or who for any other reason should not undertake muscle-tensing, should consult his or her physician before attempting any form of muscle tension therapy.

If you are in this category, you'll want to know that it is possible to skip the physical act of muscle tensing and still

198

achieve a worthwhile level of relaxation. Muscle tensing is just faster and more thorough.

•FATIGUE FIGHTER #18: Build Up Your Energy With Creative Visualization

Creative visualization is a psychological technique that enables us to create mental images for success and winning. Top coaches use it to train athletes for virtually every world class race and competitive event. Others use it to rehearse complicated gymnastic routines or swimming strokes. You can use creative visualization to improve your golf or tennis game or to help manage stress or to boost your motivation or to reinforce any of the Fatigue Fighter techniques.

FF# 17 prepares you for imagery by relaxing the body and it actually employs visualization to free your mind from all involvement with anything external. Once relaxed, you should stay on your rug or mattress and flow right on into creative imagery.

Creative visualization consists of making mental pictures of the goal you desire and reinforcing them with silent but strongly positive autogenic phrases or verbal suggestions. By combining visual symbols with verbal suggestions, we create an inner dialog that is immediately understood by both the verbally-oriented left brain and the visually-oriented right brain.

Fed into both hemispheres simultaneously, our symbols and suggestions fairly saturate the subconscious. Since the subconscious uncritically accepts all symbols and suggestions, our instructions are immediately relayed to the autonomic nervous system (ANS) to be carried out.

199

ANS nerve pathways control all involuntary functions from blood pressure to heartbeat and breathing rates, kidney function, immunity, digestion and production of enzymes and hormones.

Since the brain doesn't know the difference between a real or imagined stimulus, it responds to creative imagery by building fresh neural pathways that help us achieve whatever goal we visualize and affirm. For example, if we visualize ourself using a new and unfamiliar swimming stroke, the brain will learn, rehearse and memorize that stroke exactly as if we practiced the same stroke while in the water.

By learning to speak the language of the right brain— using symbols and imagery instead of words—our goal is communicated directly through the ANS to our involuntary functions. And whatever we have visualized or suggested gradually becomes a reality.

This powerful therapeutic tool can be used to break an addiction or unwanted habit or to create a winning attitude. Many psychologists are using it today to help treat physical or emotional problems.

Nonetheless, creative visualization is not a substitute for physical or mental action. You must still do whatever it takes to make your goal happen. But by visualizing yourself doing it, you can rehearse the scenario in your mind until you feel confident and secure that you can actually go out and do it successfully in real life.

Visualizing something is the same as creating a mental picture or making a mental image or seeing something in your mind's eye or thinking a thought. Each of us has complete personal control over our thoughts, meaning the images we hold in mind. If you doubt that, close your eyes and, for a few brief seconds, visualize first a red rose; next a snow-capped mountain peak; and finally, a dog.

Were you able to see each of these objects clearly in your mind? If so, you have the ability to visualize anything that you wish, and you also have total control over your thoughts. You are able to slide any thought (or mental picture) out of your mind and replace it with another.

And that's what you may have to do if your mind wanders while visualizing. Simply slide off the intruding thought and replace it once more with the picture you are imagining.

It's important to stay relaxed while practicing creative imagery. Avoid trying to analyze anything and don't try to force the pace. Merely maintain an attitude of passive concentration. Witness what is happening to your body while you allow your images to be absorbed. And remain open to the possibility that you will achieve your goal.

Repeat the images over and over for ten minutes at a time, once or more often each day. The more frequent and regular your imagery sessions, the sooner you should get results. As you make the mental pictures, silently repeat supporting affirmations.

The following suggestions should improve your results.

•Visualize everything as though it had already happened. Picture your adrenals as already healed and see yourself enjoying the benefits of a high-energy lifestyle. Picture your goal as if you had already achieved it. Then experience gratitude that your energy has been restored. Feel happy and fulfilled that you are now bursting with energy and experience how great life is now that you have your energy back.

•Phrase all affirmations in the present tense. Be definite and say, "I am walking five miles each day," and not "I would like to walk five miles each day." Say, "I am bursting with energy," and not "I will feel energized tomorrow." Strictly avoid phrases like, "I will be well," or "I should like to be well," or "I think I can get well," or "I want to get well," or "I will try to get well."

Employ only strong, active phrases and speak as though your goal were already accomplished: "I am doing 25 pushups each morning with ease," or "My whole body is totally re-energized." Never phrase anything in the negative, such as "I will never drink coffee again." By the same token avoid phrases like, "I won't—," or "I don't —."

•Use vivid imagery. Mentally feel, smell, hear, taste and touch everything you can in the images you visualize. Involve all your senses as you bring the picture alive. Hear the clink of your barbells as you work out. Hear the screech of gulls as they wheel overhead and feel the sand crunch under your feet as you walk briskly along a beach. Hear and feel the water hiss past your ear as you effortlessly swim. Make all your images as detailed and realistic as possible. When you visualize yourself exercising, experience how strong and energetic you feel.

•Once your images have taken hold, be willing to do what it takes to make your goals happen. The most common reason people fail to achieve their goals is that they are unwilling to do what it takes to make their goals happen.

Bearing these principles in mind, the variety of visualizations you can invent is almost limitless. You can even create images and suggestions to reinforce the effects of medication or medical treatment. However, it is usually easier to visualize a physical act than a psychological act such as restructuring a belief. To use imagery to help change your beliefs, for instance, you need to visualize it in a physical setting.

•Sample Imagery: To Reprogram a Negative Belief with a Positive Belief

Visualize yourself in a Buddhist temple in the Orient. You are barefooted and sitting crosslegged on a tatami mat floor. In front of you a candle is burning. You see a scroll lying on the floor to your left. You pick it up and unroll it. Written inside is a self-defeating belief that is causing you stress and draining your energy.

You hold the scroll over the candle and watch it burn. A black-robed priest comes forward holding an open jar. You place the ashes inside the jar. The priest withdraws with the ashes.

To your right, you see another scroll. You pick it up and unroll it. This scroll is blank. On it, using a thick marker pen, you write the new belief that will end your stress and enhance your energy.

You read the new belief over three times.

The priest reappears and takes the scroll. He tells you that the new belief is etched into your memory forever.

•Sample Imagery: To Visualize a Fatigue Fighter Technique

Fatigue Fighter #2 has already employed creative visualization to psych up your "win-power" to overcome the coffee habit. This is the same win-power that sports psychologists engender in athletes to help them win in competition.

203

FF# 3: Walk Away Fatigue, lends itself well to visualization. Let's say your goal is to briskly walk one mile along a beach each day. Begin by "feeling" charged with energy. "See" yourself dressed in shorts and T-shirt and "see" the wide, golden beach reaching away and lined by dunes. "Hear" the murmuring surf and the cries of swooping gulls overhead. And "feel" the sand crunch under your feet as you step out briskly and swing your arms. "Experience" what it feels like to walk tirelessly and with minimal effort.

Visualize scenes that best help bring your feelings of energy alive. To visualize FF# 10, see yourself turned off by foods containing sugar and white flour; instead imagine yourself enjoying brown, whole grain bread and other whole grain cereals and foods.

•Sample Imagery: Changing Your Reaction to a Potentially Stressful Life Event

Being caught each morning in a traffic jam or having to face an angry boss or the complaints of a dissatisfied customer are all triggers that may set off energy-sapping stress. Whether they do or not depends on how we perceive them and react.

Let's say your job involves dealing face-to-face with dozens of customer complaints each day. When you're run by fear-based beliefs, as most people are, it seems a natural reaction to grow weary of listening to a constant flow of criticism and dissatisfaction about your firm's products. Soon, you experience stress and begin to lose energy.

You can change this attitude by visualizing yourself in the other person's shoes and by simply witnessing the customer complaints without becoming emotionally involved. By remaining calm and seeing the other person's viewpoint, you retain the energy you need to help straighten out the customer's complaint and to do a good job for your employer. As a result, you arrive home in the evening still fresh and free of stress.

So pick the most difficult customer you encountered during the past week and to whom you reacted negatively. Visualize and re-enact the interview. But this time, avoid becoming emotionally involved. This time, simply listen without reacting to the customer's complaint and try to see things from the customer's position. Offer the customer a few words of sympathy. But stay calm and relaxed as you successfully handle the entire interview and satisfy the customer. Repeat the same scenario with other difficult customers you've interviewed recently. By visualizing yourself remaining calm and unstressed you will soon find that you remain calm and unstressed in real life.

Similar imagery can help you change your reaction to almost any potentially stressful life event.

BREAK DOWN MAJOR GOALS INTO SEVERAL EASY STEPS

To make visualizing easier, psychologists recommend dividing a major long-term goal into several short-term goals. As you succeed with the first short-term goal, positive feedback will propel you towards the next stage.

Mentally rehearse each step in a Fatigue Fighter technique and visualize yourself doing whatever it takes to achieve your goal and succeed. The end result is that an automatic process of the mind takes over and moves your muscles to achieve your goal.

Although I advise using FF# 17 to achieve deep relaxation

before flowing on into creative visualization, you can save time by using a faster relaxation method.

To relax quickly, lie down, close your eyes and watch and listen to your breathing. Take slow, deep breaths. Feel yourself relaxing with each exhalation. Feel the tension flowing out of your right leg as you exhale a breath. On the next exhalation, feel the tension leave your left leg. With each succeeding exhalation, mentally drain the tension from your abdomen, chest and shoulders, arms, neck and face. With a few deep breaths you can be completely relaxed. Then slide into creative visualization.

Even though your mental pictures do not appear to be vivid and clear, they will inevitably work. However, if you have trouble imagining, you can make clearer images by writing out your affirmations.

To do this, you must relax in a chair instead of lying down. Then, instead of silently saying the affirmations, write them over and over on a sheet of paper. The act of writing stimulates powerful imagery in almost everyone.

One caution: anyone with an emotional or mental disorder, or who experiences hallucinations, should consult his or her personal physician before using visualization.

By using the temple scene for belief reprogramming described earlier, you can visualize yourself acting out—and succeeding with—virtually every Fatigue Fighter in this book.

•FATIGUE FIGHTER #18-A: Using Cognitive Positivism to Restructure Worn-Out Beliefs That Are Destroying Your Energy

Most people's minds are run by a block of fear-based beliefs called the *ego* or *lower mind*. The ego is that part of the mind concerned with the nurturing, comfort, procreation and survival of the body. It's our animal nature. And it sees as hostile anything that it believes might threaten our security, prestige, comfort or pleasure.

By distorting the rational thinking process, the ego causes people to perceive hostility and unfriendliness where none may exist. Working at the University of Pennsylvania Medical School some years ago, David D. Burns, M.D., discovered that most cases of psychologically caused depression are created, not by some complex biochemical process deep within the body, but by ten common types of illogical thinking.

Curiously, almost all of us are quite familiar with these irrational ways of using the mind. Distorted thinking ranges from making a mountain out a molehill to exaggerating a minor drawback while ignoring an overwhelming number of advantages. It includes "all or nothing" thinking—seeing yourself as a total failure if your performance falls short in merely one area even though you have succeeded everywhere else. Many people also allow themselves to be run by the way they feel: "This feels bad, therefore it must be bad." Again, prefacing statements with "must," "ought," "should" or "shouldn't" is an almost guaranteed way to twist around your thinking.

Dr. Burns discovered that these, and similar variations of distorted thinking, are responsible for most depression and anxiety. By getting depressed patients to recognize that the cause of their problem is the irrational ways in which they use their minds, Dr. Burns perfected a do-it-yourself method for reversing depression. He called it Cognitive Therapy.

It works by teaching a depressed person to identify the ten

variations of distorted thinking, and to learn to think once more in a rational way. When this happens, most cases of depression and angst disappear.

Since Dr. Burns' discovery, other researchers have shown that irrational thinking is also associated with holding negative beliefs. Meanwhile, yet another school of therapy has grown out of the principle of Positive Thinking first developed by Dr. Norman Vincent Peale.

By putting it all together—Cognitive Therapy plus Belief Restructuring plus Positive Thinking—we come up with Cognitive Positivism, the most powerful healing tool in the entire field of behavioral medicine.

By combining the power of all three psychotherapies, Cognitive Positivism straightens out distorted thinking by replacing inappropriate, energy-destroying beliefs with positive, energy-enhancing affirmations. And instead of continuing to be anxious or depressed, a person begins to see the world in a friendly, positive way that eventually leads to lasting happiness, satisfaction and fulfillment.

Without going into any more detail, if you have chronic tiredness and it's caused by depression or anxiety, and your doctor can find no physical cause, then Cognitive Positivism may well be the answer to your chronic fatigue.

To begin using Cognitive Positivism, you should first use FF# 17 to enter a state of deep relaxation. (Or you may use the accelerated relaxation technique described at the end of FF# 18.)

All you need do then is to accept, one by one, each of the positive beliefs listed below. Starting with number one, study each belief until you have accepted it completely. Use creative visualization to see yourself bestow forgiveness on each person whom you believe may have caused you harm at some time. Visualize yourself forgiving one person a. time—and don't forget to forgive yourself as well. Totally accept each belief, and absorb it, before going on to the next belief.

Naturally, you should first read and memorize each belief you plan to accept before you enter deep relaxation. By the simple act of mentally accepting each new love-based belief, you will also be releasing its opposite, the fear-based belief that is the cause of your stress and your chronic fatigue.

Ten Positive Affirmations For Restructuring Your Belief System

1. I forgive and release forever anyone I have not for-given—including myself. I forgive everyone, everything and every circumstance, totally and *right now*. Nor do I expect to be always treated with fairness and justice. Both exist only in my mind and I am immediately ready to forgive anyone whom my ego may "see" as unfair or unjust. For I know that unforgiveness is a major underlying cause of cancer and other diseases and is one of the primary causes of chronic fatigue.

2. I know there is nothing to fear. I absolutely refuse to waste energy worrying about the future or lamenting the past. All fears about the future exist only in my imagination and are pure fantasy. I am a powerful person and I am completely capable of handling whatever the future may bring. Besides, when it arrives, the future will have become the present. I also totally let go of the past and with it, all guilt and resentment.

3. I love everyone unconditionally, including and espe-cially myself. I accept everyone the way they are without

209

requiring them to change. I experience a deep one-ness with all other people and living things. I refuse to see myself as separate from others. When I meet another person, especially of another race or culture, I look for the similarities between us, not for the differences. Whether in thought, word or deed, I cease to judge, criticize, condemn or attack another person. I see only the best in everyone, including myself. To do otherwise is to create a constant drain on my energy.

4. I am always optimistic, hopeful, cheerful and positive. I expect good things to happen to me today, tomorrow and throughout life. I practice positivism every moment of the day. I accept all the warmth and joy in life but I allow negativity to flow past me and I simply witness it without reacting. To be here is joy, to exist is bliss, to be alive is sheer happiness. Joy, bliss and happiness are my birthright and I can enjoy them constantly unless I allow a fear-based belief or thought to enter my mind. Thus there is no room in my mind for depression or anxiety, the promoters of chronic tiredness.

5. I am healing myself! I am a high-energy person! For healing is to let go of fear and fear-based beliefs. I am completely healed, I can't be sick. My birthright is perfect health and unlimited energy. My normal state is to be a high-energy person. So every day in every way I have more and more energy.

6. I do and acquire only things that will maintain and deepen my inner peace. I cease craving superficial excitement and stimulation. I recognize that lasting happiness, satisfaction and fulfillment come only from contentment and not from things that I do, buy, eat or drink. I am content to be wherever I am here and now. I always have everything I need to enjoy the present moment, therefore my needs and

wants are few. Only when I am calm, centered and serene do I make choices and decisions. I avoid acting or choosing when I feel emotionally upset. When I am content and at ease, and my body and mind are still and relaxed, my energy level begins to soar.

7. I think in terms of cooperation rather than competition. I can only win where everyone wins. I also share the good and success that comes to others without experiencing envy. I never compare myself with others or with their accomplishments or possessions. As a result, I am liberated from envy. And I will further conserve my energy by enjoying every moment of every day regardless of where I am, how I'm feeling, who I'm with or what I'm doing.

8. I experience only abundance and I am willing to share my abundance with others. For I realize that giving and receiving are the same. Whatever I give or lose, I will receive back several times over. I also recognize that absolute material security is unattainable. Yet I know that I will always have what I need when I need it. I also act without anticipating results, without seeking the fruits or rewards of my actions. I have no desire for praise, attention, fame or recognition nor to appear publicly important. I will not do anything merely to win the approval of others. I refuse to experience pride and I always practice humility. This helps me avoid disappointment, another common energy drain. (Note: these principles do not apply to gambling or betting nor to "loaning" money to financially-irresponsible people, including members of your own family.)

9. I view each of life's seeming problems as a challenge and as a fresh opportunity to grow, to progress and to learn, and not as a fight against the clock or against another person or another corporation. I also accept complete responsibility

for my life and for everything that happens to me. By seeing problems as a learning experience, they become energy boosters instead of energy drains.

10. I am a hardy person. I am not intimidated by minor discomforts or inconveniences nor by physical or mental exertion. I am completely willing to step outside my comfort zone. I never give up or give in. I always act as if it is impossible to fail. Thus my mind has no room for such energy-destroying beliefs as: "Exercise is work or punishment; I'll never be any good at exercise (or tennis, etc.); I don't have the time or the energy to exercise; I feel deprived if I can't eat lots of fat and meat."

COGNITIVE POSITIVISM TO THE RESCUE

Cognitive Positivism changes the way you feel by changing the way you believe and think. It does so by having you replace old, worn-out conditioned beliefs—which you acquired in the distant past—with new positive beliefs which are more appropriate to your present lifestyle.

A typical conditioned belief, still held by millions of men and women, is "I never forgive a slight." Fear-based beliefs of this type were frequently conditioned into us during childhood or perhaps in school, or in the armed forces or by teachers, parents or other people. In past years, some of these beliefs might have had some validity. But their usefulness has long been outlived.

To perceive life through a filter of conditioned beliefs today is to see a world that is threatening and hostile when, in reality, it is perfectly harmless and safe. The result: your stress mechanisms are turned on and your energy is depleted.

Cognitive Positivism functions automatically when you adopt and absorb the ten love-based affirmations just listed. These powerfully positive and expansive beliefs so fill your mind that no space remains for old, outdated beliefs based on fear.

The result is to liberate you from stress. And in the process depression, anxiety and chronic fatigue become just a memory.

CHAPTER TWELVE

Ten Ways to
Fatigue-Proof
Your Life

Few people seem willing to trade our modern hi-tech, industrialized culture for a simpler lifestyle. But it is largely the effects of our modern lifestyle that are responsible for the current epidemic of chronic fatigue.

Extensive daily physical exercise and muscular exertion are essential biological needs if people are to remain healthy and vigorous. But when they surrender all opportunity for using their muscles to machines and appliances, it's no wonder that their energy mechanisms shut down. Add in hours each day of watching other people lead active lives on a TV screen while passively sitting and doing nothing, and it's hardly surprising that millions of people have lost the ability to tap into their energy resources.

Meanwhile, the pressures of trying to work and survive in urban America are often so stressful that they place a constant drain on whatever energy remains.

Chronic tiredness is almost entirely lifestyle associated. Yet we don't *have* to lose our health and energy to survive. We can still function in, and enjoy the benefits of modern living, without being destroyed.

The solution is this. Put together, the 18 Fatigue Fighter techniques in this book form an alternative lifestyle through which you can virtually fatigue-proof yourself. First, the Fatigue Fighters help you to avoid most of the pitfalls and traps of modern living that sap your energy. Then, by simply dropping each of your energy-destroying habits and replacing it with an energy-boosting behavior, the Fatigue Fighters create a completely fatigue-proof way to live.

It's patently obvious that our culture encourages people to eat more and more high-fat high-sugar foods, to exercise less and less, and to go into debt to buy more and more things that only end up increasing the stress in their lives.

Thus to re-energize yourself, you need to do exactly the opposite. By making the Fatigue Fighters a permanent part of your lifestyle, you can become a high-energy person able to live and thrive in a fatigue-inducing culture.

If you've read this book so far, you'll realize that most of the habits, foods, beliefs and other lifestyle factors that enhance your energy have already been covered in previous chapters. So the purpose of this chapter is to review ten other energy-enriching steps, each of which can help to fatigue-proof your life.

*STEP I. Restructure Your Time and Invest in Yourself for a Change

In these days of dual income families, few people can spare the time to even microwave dinner, let alone to exercise, visualize, or meditate. Yet to rebuild your energy you must create sufficient time to practice the Fatigue Fighter techniques.

The place to begin may be right in your living room. As you'll read in Step 2, most people spend at least 2½ hours daily watching TV—a total of 17½ hours each week. Cut out TV watching altogether and you'll have an entire extra day of free time each week.

Additionally, consider cutting out any activity that isn't genuinely productive, essential or worthwhile. Certainly, performing volunteer work can empower you and bolster your self-esteem. Yet you should never allow all your free time to be devoted to the benefit of others, leaving no time at all to nurture and care for the health of your own body and mind.

Everyone today has too much to do and too little time to do it in. That's why popping a tranquilizer seems so much easier than taking time to stretch, breathe deeply and practice deep relaxation. But that's just one of many lifetraps that lie in wait to ensnare us.

So prune away all non-essential activities. For example, plan ahead so that you don't have to stand in line at the bank or supermarket during the Friday afternoon crush. Go on Wednesday instead. Shop early in the morning or after 8:00 p.m., when supermarkets are often empty. Plan all activities well in advance so that you start out in plenty of time, especially for work. Find the location of any new place you must visit on a street map before leaving home.

Even out your workweek by spreading your chores and workload evenly over each day. Many of us could gradually phase out a busy schedule by pacing ourselves differently. Define your real goals and priorities and eliminate all trivia or activities that fritter away your time and don't really contribute to your life or anyone else's.

Above all, schedule your daily exercise routine ahead of almost everything else. Exercise should be a deliberately-planned activity—as essential as sleeping or eating—and not the last thing on your list. So try to make it your number one priority.

Never allow lack of equipment or inability to go outdoors to stop you from exercising. You can do scores of different calisthenics and stretching exercises on the living room floor and then run or step in place without needing anything in the way of equipment. And never put off exercising because you must work out by yourself.

If you seem overburdened by activities, drop all or most of your time-consuming minor obligations. Then avoid filling your calender with appointments and don't commit yourself to deadlines and schedules that are not absolutely vital.

Instead, select a quiet, unstructured period each day for a walk among trees and grass and become aware of the sky and clouds and the sounds, shapes, moods and colors of nature. If you are unable to do this at least several times a week, you may be pursuing inappropriate goals.

Or, are you working ten hours a day so that you can rush through life and have a heart attack in a few years? If so, learn now to say "no" to relatives or other people who make excessive demands on your time. Avoid getting trapped into

217

participating in community or voluntary activities that require a heavy work load.

Finally, try to avoid spending disproportionate amounts of time chauffeuring your children around. When conditions are safe, children are well able to walk one or two miles or to bicycle longer distances. Alternatively, work out a carpooling arrangement and share the driving with other parents.

•STEP 2. Break TV Addiction—The Great Energy Drain

Watching TV can be as addictive as a drug. Surveys show that the average American spends at least 2½ hours daily in a mindless stupor hypnotized by a babbling TV tube. A sedentary person who watches TV all evening is likely to be tired all the time, since TV viewing is totally passive, both physically and mentally.

Most programs overstimulate the mind, causing it to continue running at full speed long after you switch off the set. Many of the commercials brainwash you into eating junk foods that impede your energy mechanisms. And the majority of programs keep your level of tension and anxiety high while effectively destroying your imagination, creativity, energy and health and those of your children as well.

When Professor Larry A. Tucker, Ph.D., Director of Health Promotion at Brigham Young University in Provo, Utah, studied the viewing habits and fitness levels of 9,000 adults, he found that the fittest people watched TV for less than one hour each day. Those who watched for three to four hours daily were 41 percent less fit and those who watched for four hours or more were 50 percent less fit. A similar study of 800 adults, published in the *Journal of the American Dietetic Association* in 1990, reported that while only 4.5 percent of people who watched TV for one hour or less daily were obese, the percentage of obese individuals rose to 19.2 percent among those who watched the tube for four hours or more each day.

Is your energy being sapped because you are a TV junkie?

If you watch the screen for more than two hours daily, and if you become irritated or unhappy when you cannot watch it, you may well be addicted to television.

Helping to confirm TV addiction are the following symptoms. You snack on junk food and sip beer or soft drinks while watching TV. You watch TV while lying awake in bed during periods of sleeplessness. You switch on the TV set as soon as you enter a room and, even though you have no definite program to watch, you scan the channels to find an entertaining program. On a fine, sunny day, you prefer to stay indoors and watch television rather than to enjoy some form of recreation out of doors. Anyone who fits this TV-junkie profile is also likely to be overweight, unfit and suffering from poor nutrition, insomnia and chronic fatigue.

To start weaning yourself from TV, go through the TV section in the Sunday paper. Mark only programs that make you laugh or that are inspirational, educational or documentaries. Allow yourself an average of only one hour of viewing each day. Watch only these shows and turn off the TV at all other times. Instead, read or take up a new hobby or sign up for a new class or go outdoors and garden, walk, bicycle, swim or exercise at a gym.

Better yet, watch only Public Television or the Discovery

Channel. Both feature splendid documentaries on the fine arts, nature, the sciences and the environment. Next best are funny movies or comedy programs. Spurn all shows that feature violence: they create unrealistic fears about crime and your safety. Instead of watching sports and ball games, become a participant in an active game such as tennis or volleyball. Also, avoid watching late night talk shows and news programs. Both can be disturbing and cause sleep difficulties.

To minimize stress while watching a program, sit at least eight feet away from the set and keep a dim light on to reduce eyestrain and stimulation. During commercials, stand up and walk around or do some stretches or other exercises. Never eat for entertainment while watching TV and avoid conversing during a program. As soon as the program ends, switch off the set and take a brisk walk outdoors.

As with other addictions, the most successful solution is often to quit watching TV altogether. This one decision may do more to end chronic tiredness and to improve your life than any other single thing you can do.

•STEP 3. Spend Time with High-Energy People

To become a high-energy person, seek out the company of high-energy people. Observe how they eat, think and operate and model your lifestyle on theirs. Stay strictly away from anyone who smokes, has an alcohol problem or uses drugs. Mix, instead, with health-conscious people who eat natural foods and who exercise and lead active, meaningful lives.

To do this may mean giving up old acquaintances who always seem tired. Though this may sound cruel, the fact is that many low-energy people drain the energy of those

220

around them. It's particularly exhausting to listen to someone with a victim complex who is continually describing how he or she has been exploited or abused. You may also want to drop family members in this category. Instead of allowing them to drag you down to their level, begin loving yourself by eating right and exercising.

All too often, the main problem with upgrading your diet is social. You can't find healthful foods in most restaurants and at family or social events you must eat what you're served. By associating instead with health-conscious people, you avoid this problem entirely.

•STEP 4. Beat Boredom by Becoming an Exciting and Energetic Person

If you drag yourself through the day's work, then perk up at quitting time, you have situational fatigue. You are fatigued only in certain situations and the cause is invariably boredom.

Experts have predicted that every day 50 million Americans are severely bored with their jobs or with housework or other routine chores. But as soon as they switch to an exciting or stimulating activity, their fatigue vanishes. While situational fatigue is a temporary condition, if allowed to persist, it can turn into chronic tiredness.

The solution is to transform boredom into excitement and to make routine tasks more enjoyable. Housekeeping chores become much more enjoyable, for instance, when you turn on some music and make vacuuming and sweeping a part of your exercise program.

A sudden bit of serendipity or a burst of laughter can

221

banish boredom in seconds. Both acts release hormones called catecholamines that can swiftly transform fatigue into a condition of excitement and high energy.

To get yourself excited about life, choose two activities or goals that really turn you on. For instance, choose a hobby or recreation that you've always wanted to do. Few people can change their jobs, so the next best thing is to build interest and excitement outside your work.

These goals could range from getting married to jumping off a bungie tower to learning to use a computer with new software or cooking exotic dishes or solving challenging puzzles. To help plan an exciting future, check out library books and begin to build a dream project in one of your chosen fields.

By becoming involved in an absorbing activity, you will quickly dispel the aimlessness and drifting-along and the playing-everything-safe attitude that makes for boredom. Instead, plan an adventurous future and be prepared to take a few mild risks. For example, you might take up an entirely new sport or activity even though you may not do it well. Or you could become an environmental or political activist and risk controversy.

Exactly what your goals are is up to you; they could include dressmaking, home remodeling, decorating, gardening or health improvement. Whatever it is, choose something upbeat, especially if it brings you into contact with others. If you experience museum fatigue in an art gallery, consider taking a course in art history and appreciation.

Regardless of your age or occupation, you can become an exciting and energetic person when you overcome boredom and situational fatigue.

•STEP 5. Breathe Pure Air Whenever You Can

An abundance of pure oxygen is essential for efficient functioning of the energy mechanism. Studies have shown that people who inhale smog and polluted air tire much more easily than they otherwise would. Constant exposure to polluted air causes the cells in the lungs to thicken and die while the lungs lose elasticity and the ability to exchange carbon dioxide for oxygen.

When people seal their homes and workplaces against outdoor pollution, or against cold weather, this also creates a low oxygen level. As you breathe and consume oxygen in the indoor air, no fresh air flows in to replace it. During winter, millions of American homes and workplaces have a dangerously low oxygen level that weakens people's energy.

For those who live in polluted cities like Los Angeles, part of chronic tiredness could be due to lung damage caused by polluted air. But whenever the air outdoors is pure, it's up to you to open the windows and bring in a supply of fresh, oxygen-laden air.

•STEP 6. Take Short, Frequent Rests

Recent work studies have found that on-the-job fatigue can be dramatically reduced by taking short, frequent rests that ideally total ten minutes every hour.

One study showed that two five-minute breaks each hour for seven days provided more refreshment and renewal than working six days and taking an entire day off.

For maximum benefit, spend your break of five minutes or longer outside the workplace and preferably outdoors.

223

Failing that, sit down, close your eyes and visualize yourself in a beautiful natural setting (see FF#18).

Of course, you don't have to be at work to benefit from frequent rests. Regardless of what kind of activity you're doing, schedule at least two five-minute breaks each hour.

•STEP 7. Tap Your Body's Circadian Energy Rhythms

A mix of circadian rhythms regulate our levels of energy and alertness, hunger, temperature and even mood. Most people experience an overall low in body rhythms between 3:00 a.m. and 5:00 a.m. when hormone levels are depressed, heart rate slows and body temperature drops by as much as two degrees. From then on, hormone levels and temperature gradually rise, reaching a peak later in the morning or even in midafternoon.

These rhythms explain why many people feel sluggish early in the morning and may not reach peak performance until as late as 4:00 p.m. These rhythms may also be influenced by drugs, beverages, sleep habits, food and, particularly, by the time of day you exercise.

This last is the clue to boosting your energy by influencing your circadian rhythms. Assuming you walk briskly for exercise, you can be at peak alertness and arousal by scheduling your walk some two hours earlier. For example, to have your energy peak at 9:00 a.m., you should take a brisk 30-minute walk at around 6:30 a.m. Exercising to this schedule helps overcome any midmorning "low" and it supplies an endorphin "high" just as you arrive at work.

Likewise, to experience maximum energy and alertness at 3:00 p.m., you should schedule a brisk walk during your lunch hour. By warming up the body you also warm up the

224

mind. For this same reason, it's best to avoid walking after 7:00 p.m. Otherwise, you'll reach your energy peak just before bedtime and be unable to fall asleep.

•STEP 8. Avoid Creating Potential Stress in Your Life

Endeavor to avoid potentially stressful life events and, as far as is possible, leave them entirely out of your lifestyle.

For starters, avoid going into debt, especially to buy something—a new car or home, for instance—because you believe that possessing it will bring you lasting happiness. Buying a new car may lift your spirits for a week or two but once you must face the burdensome monthly payments and the astronomical insurance premiums, the net result is more likely to be long-term stress than long-term happiness.

Most Americans have already mortgaged almost all their disposable income for two to three years ahead. Should an emergency occur, they must borrow again. Having to meet debt payments is one of the most widespread causes of stress in America. Yet millions of Americans could cut their stress levels in half by postponing the purchase of consumer goods until they were able to pay with cash.

Try to avoid becoming a workaholic or having to work under excessive pressure or competition or in a workplace with a demanding boss. The most stressful jobs are those on the lowest rungs of the ladder: dead-end jobs like waitress or laborer that leave no choices, options or alternatives. Chronic fatigue is twice as common among workers in dead-end jobs as in those able to exercise some autonomy and control.

Again, many women who are homemakers experience

anger or depression because they feel they are not out working and making a contribution. Meanwhile, millions of employed women are equally angry and stressed because they
must do housework and care for children after spending the
day at the office.

It's mainly the prolonged stresses, those with little relief in
sight, that lead to depression and chronic tiredness. Among
the most stressful life events are retirement, unemployment,
the burden of caring for aging parents, loss of money or
possessions, divorce or separation, or becoming a parent.

To help avoid chronic tiredness, consider turning down
any request asking you to do something that causes repeated
stress. Set a pace for your life that you can stay with. Identify
your priorities, do only things that are really essential, and
give yourself a long, daily leisure break. Use it to enjoy
music, to read, to exercise or to play games outdoors. And
avoid planning ambitious, fast-paced vacations, or days off,
that fill your leisure time with targets and goals.

List the most stressful situations in your life and give top
priority to ameliorating them or getting them out of your life
entirely.

If you should experience stress, use this quick-action step
to release it immediately.

A FAST-ACTION STEP TO IMMEDIATELY RELEASE STRESS

1. Keep on breathing smoothly and steadily but take
deeper breaths and inhale more air.
2. Smile—even if you don't feel like it. The act of smiling

relaxes every muscle in your eyes, lips and face and induces relaxation in the rest of your body.

3. Quickly visualize yourself hanging suspended from a hook in the top of your head. Drop your shoulders and let your entire spine and body hang loose, relaxed and straight.

4. Swiftly scan your body for any sign of muscle tension. If you locate a tension-filled muscle, deliberately tense that muscle briefly for six seconds and release.

5. Imagine a wave of relaxation wafting down over your entire body and washing away all tension, leaving you wonderfully calm and relaxed.

6. Immediately forgive the person or circumstance that triggered the stress. Never deny that stress is occuring. Instead, perceive it as nonthreatening. Witness it without reacting. Avoid becoming emotionally involved with what is causing it. Tell yourself that by remaining calm and detached, you are much better able to solve the problem.

•STEP 9. Dealing with Fatigue Due to Seasonal Affective Disorder

More commonly known as "cabin fever," Seasonal Affective Disorder (SAD) is, nonetheless, a well-documented cause of depression and fatigue during the winter months. It is a light-sensitive form of depression caused by insufficient light to trigger the release of hormones in the brain that keep people feeling good. And, of course, it is most common in the northern states where gloomy, overcast weather blocks out the sun during the winter months.

In our northern states, SAD is a common cause of seasonal fatigue. According to the National Institute of Mental

Health, literally millions of Americans are affected by SAD. Eighty-three percent are women aged 30 to 50. And the gender difference is because fewer women go outdoors during the winter months.

The cure for SAD-induced fatigue is easy. You simply need to go outdoors and expose your eyes and body to natural, full-spectrum daylight for an hour or more each day. So go outdoors and exercise regularly during the day. It also helps to open up window shades and drapes and bring more daylight into your home.

The sun doesn't have to be shining when you go outdoors. The clouds allow enough full-spectrum light through to lift your depression and dispel your fatigue.

•STEP 10. Learn to Increase Your Sexual Energy

"Not tonight, honey. I'm too tired."

Deciding to take a rain check on one of life's most exciting and enjoyable pleasures may not always be due to physical tiredness or to lack of energy. For instance, the actual amount of energy expended in a full hour of torrid lovemaking seldom exceeds that needed to walk up six flights of stairs.

Yet mobilizing energy for sex is a complex process that involves just about every function of the energy mechanisms described in this book. And as you may suspect, it often has more to do with loss of psychological desire than with actual lack of physical energy.

Stress and depression, two factors frequently associated with chronic tiredness, are primarily responsible for lowering sexual appetite. Both influence the central nervous system to decrease the body's supply of testosterone. This sex hormone is produced in both men and women and is needed by both to build sexual desire. Studies have shown that, while under stress, men often show a dramatic decline in testosterone levels. When depressed or under stress, sex is the last thing most people think about.

Among other psychological reasons cited by therapists for avoiding sex is fear of an inferior performance, and fear that close intimacy may put a person under an obligation to give more time to the relationship that would add pressure to an already tight schedule. The sex drive may also be impaired by alcohol, smoking, some birth control pills or OTC diet pills, and by certain prescription drugs, particularly anti-hypertensive medications.

Whether inability to become aroused and experience sexual pleasure is actually due to chronic tiredness, or to a psychological cause, the following steps may help to rekindle desire and to mobilize the energy needed to enjoy active sex.

1. Give lovemaking a higher priority on your value scale. Don't leave it until bedtime when your energy may actually be waning. By making love on weekend mornings, or during the day, your creativity and imagination are also likely to be more active. Some couples schedule lovemaking several days in advance and both write down dates and times.

2. Besides hugging, kissing and touching, an important part of satisfying sex for women is the revealing of deep feelings. Exchanging such intimate confidences is often difficult for men. Yet for many women, learning of their partner's feelings can contribute more to a perfect sex experience than actual intercourse.

3. Each partner should take an active role in initiating sex. It shouldn't all be left up to the man.

4. Lovemaking is impossible unless both partners go to

229

bed at the same time. You can't expect satisfying sex if you stay up while your spouse goes to bed. And if you're both in the mood, watching TV prior to lovemaking can quickly destroy those special feelings. Smoking or drinking alcohol prior to lovemaking may also kill the sex drive. Cigarette smoke constricts arteries in the penis, weakening an erection, while alcohol inhibits release of most sex hormones, making it difficult to climax.

All of these are actually motivation strategies. As with most other activities, once you develop the required motivation, the bodymind supplies all the energy you need—whether it's for making love or exercising or cleaning the house or meeting an emergency—even if you *have* had a tiring day.

GLOSSARY

Active Therapy. A treatment in which the patient plays an active role in his or her own recovery. Typical active therapies include exercise, relaxation, upgrading the diet and nutrition, and using creative visualization or cognitive positivism.

Adrenal Glands. A pair of endocrine glands, one atop each kidney, that secrete hormones that regulate key functions of the energy process. (See under "Adrenal burnout" in Chapter 4.)

Aerobic Exercise. A continuous, rhythmic movement that uses the body's large muscle groups for a prolonged period at a speed which raises the rate of both pulse and breathing. Aerobic exercise is supplied by brisk walking, bicycling, jogging, swimming, dancing or cross-country skiing. These exercises use the body's slow-twitch muscles, which results in increased oxygen uptake and strengthening and toning of the entire cardiovascular system.

Amino Acids. The building blocks of protein, which forms the tissue, cells, bones, nerves, muscles and organs of the body. Of the total 22 amino acids, the body can

231

synthesize only 13. The remaining 9—called Essential Amino Acids—must be obtained directly from the diet.

Anaerobic Exercise. Exercise such as weight-lifting or pole-vaulting which uses the fast-twitch muscles for short bursts of energy without much need for oxygen. Anaerobic exercise fails to build up the heart or lungs or to benefit the energy mechanism.

Anxiety or Angst. Worrying or fear about a possibility of loss at some future time.

Apnea. A sleep-disturbing dysfunction common among overweight, middle-aged men which frequently causes chronic fatigue.

ATP (Adenosine Triphosphate). Before it can actually fuel a muscle, glucose must be transformed into ATP. For this to occur, sufficient creatinine phosphate and co-enzyme Q-10 (ubiquinine) must be present. Only three ounces of ATP can exist in the body at any given moment, enough to sustain a runner for only six or seven seconds.

Autogenic Phrases. Verbal suggestions or affirmations which are repeated silently to reinforce a goal visualized during creative visualization. Autogenic phrases may also be silently repeated at other times.

Aversion Therapy. A do-it-yourself psychological technique for breaking addictions. (See FF#2-A.)

Behavioral Medicine. The branch of medicine based on changing the way people feel by the way they act or behave. In behavioral therapy, action must precede motivation and healing. This philosophy ensures that people take an active role in their own recovery.

Belief Restructuring. Straightening out distorted thinking by replacing self-defeating beliefs with positive, health-enhancing beliefs.

Carbohydrate Loading. Eating a diet high in complex carbohydrates for several days prior to an athletic event to
ensure that, by the time of the event, the liver and
muscles are loaded with glycogen.

Carbohydrates, Complex. Complex carbohydrates are found
in fruits, vegetables, whole grains, legumes, seeds,
sprouts and nuts in the same unprocessed and unrefined
state in which they grow in nature. When digested,
these plant-based foods become glucose, the preferred
energy source for the brain and muscles. Complex carbohydrates are high in fiber, low in fat and bestow many
health benefits. They are also known as "good" carbohydrates. Because the sugars and starches in complex carbohydrates are enclosed in cellulose or fiber, they are
slowly released into the bloodstream; this maintains a
stable blood sugar level.

Carbohydrates, Simple or Refined. Simple carbohydrates
usually consist of wheat, sugar or rice that has been
refined into white flour, white sugar or white rice. Refining strips these foods of much of their beneficial fiber
and other nutrients, leaving little more than empty calories. Refined carbohydrates are often called "bad" carbohydrates, yet they constitute one-fifth of all food eaten
by the average American.

Catecholamines. Consisting of three hormones—adrenalin,
noradrenalin and dopamine—catecholamines control
the fight or flight response.

Chronic Fatigue Syndrome (CFS), also known as **Chronic
Fatigue Immune Deficiency Syndrome (CFIDS).** A
documented disease condition believed to arise from a
virus attack on the immune system in which the principle symptom is chronic fatigue. CFS is described in

233

detail under "Step 5: Eliminate Chronic Fatigue Syndrome" in Chapter 2.

Chronic Tiredness. Chronic tiredness is a state of constant weariness, fatigue or near-exhaustion which is symptomatic of an underlying condition. Approximately 80 percent of chronic tiredness appears to be due to such underlying lifestyle causes as sleep deprivation, sedentary living, poor diet or unresolved emotional stress, while the remaining 20 percent appears due to an underlying physical or psychological disease or dysfunction or to the adverse side effects of OTC or prescription drugs. The condition known as chronic tiredness differs from the immuno-viral disease called Chronic Fatigue Syndrome (see above). Chronic tiredness is a mindbody, or whole-person, condition that requires a holistic or whole-person approach to overcome.

Co-enzyme Q-10 (ubiquinine). A substance essential in the biochemical transformation of glucose into ATP (adenosine triphosphate), the actual fuel which powers the muscles. A deficiency of co-enzyme Q-10 may lead to lethargy and chronic tiredness.

Cognitive Positivism. Often considered the most powerful tool in behavioral medicine, cognitive positivism is a combination of cognitive therapy, belief restructuring and positive thinking.

Cognitive Therapy. This psychological healing tool teaches a person to identify the ten variations of distorted thinking and to learn to think once more in a rational way. When this happens, most cases of psychologically-caused anxiety and depression fade away.

Creatinine Phosphate (CP). CP is a key substance in transforming glucose into ATP (adenosine triphosphate), the actual fuel which energizes the muscles.

Creative Visualization or **Creative Imagery**. Making mental pictures of the goal you desire and reinforcing these images with silent but strongly positive autogenic phrases (verbal suggestions or affirmations).

Depression. A major cause of inertia, an attitude which effectively blocks the body's energy mechanisms from functioning efficiently.

Clinical Depression is a serious personality syndrome in which a person often feels hopeless, helpless, worthless and pessimistic and may contemplate suicide. All such cases are major depressive disorders and require treatment by a psychologist or psychiatrist.

Chronic Low Grade Depression is a milder but persistant form of depression characterized by low energy levels, fatigue and poor self-esteem.

Mild Depression is normally not serious enough to require antidepressants or psychiatric counseling and it often responds well to Cognitive Therapy. Nonetheless, one of its symptoms may be chronic fatigue.

Cool-Down. Reducing speed to a relaxed pace at the end of a walk or aerobic workout, then stretching the muscles used in exercising to prevent pooling of blood in the legs and a sudden rise in blood pressure.

Deep Muscle Relaxation. A combination of both physical and psychological techniques designed to replace neuro-muscular tension with a deep level of relaxation.

Endorphins. The body's own natural narcotics that block pain receptors in the brain and make you feel good. Endorphins are released by brisk exercise or by thinking positively.

Energy Mechanism. The body's energy mechanism is actually a series of systems and mechanisms that break down food into glucose to energize the muscles and brain.

235

Fat is also used as a second choice muscle fuel. The adrenal and thyroid glands control energy production while the fight or flight response makes energy instantly available in an emergency.

Epstein-Barr Virus. Fatigue is a major symptom of this fairly common viral disorder, which is also the primary cause of mononucleosis. See "Other Common Fatigue-Causing Diseases" in Chapter 2.

Fast-Twitch Muscles. Fast-twitch muscles respond quickly to provide short bursts of energy for such anaerobic exercises as weight-lifting or pole-vaulting.

Fat. Compared to glucose from carbohydrate foods, fat is a poor fuel for body muscles. The body itself prefers to draw on glucose to power the muscles and turns to fat only as a second choice fuel when glucose supplies run low. You can increase your energy and improve your health by eating twice as much complex carbohydrates as fat.

Fibromyalgia or **Fibrositis.** A common cause of chronic tiredness, fibromyalgia primarily affects women aged 20 to 50. See "Other Common Fatigue-Causing Diseases" in Chapter 2.

Fight or Flight Response. The body's emergency arousal state, triggered by the mind whenever it perceives a situation—whether real or imagined—as threatening or hostile. For as long as the response continues to simmer, it stresses the adrenal glands and drains the body's energy resources. (See Chapter 4.)

Generalization of Effect. The psychologist's term for the phenomenon in which a natural ability to succeed in one field can be transferred to a less successful area of life. One may then achieve equal success in the second field.

236

Glucocorticosteroid Hormones. These hormones, principally cortisol, control the metabolism of food into energy. Others regulate muscle integrity and control mineral balance.

Glucose. A form of sugar which fuels body muscles. Glucose is produced when starches and sugars in plant-based foods (carbohydrates) are broken down and digested. Until required for use, surplus glucose is stored in the liver and muscles as glycogen.

Gut-Feeling Scale. A subjective method of estimating the pulse rate while exercising by how hard the exercise feels.

GTF—Glucose Tolerance Factor. A complex molecule that, in optimal amounts, ensures higher energy levels by helping to regulate the blood sugar level and by improving the synthesis and storage of glycogen in liver and muscles.

Heart Rate Target Zone. By keeping your pulse rate within this zone while exercising aerobically, training effect can be achieved without overdoing it. To calculate your personal heart rate target zone, subtract your age from 220. The result is your maximum heart rate or "max." Your heart rate target zone lies between 60 and 80 percent of max.

Heme. One of two forms of dietary iron, heme forms hemoglobin and exists only in foods of animal origin.

Hi-Carb Diet. For optimal performance, most athletes today eat a high-carbohydrate diet which supplies protein plus fiber and energy, not merely protein plus fat as is the case with most meat and dairy products. A diet high in complex carbohydrates is the best source of readily-available energy for aerobic exercise.

Holistic Medicine, or **Holistic Healing.** Holistic medicine uses an array of natural (and sometimes also medical) therapies that function on all levels of the bodymind, employing a multi-level, multi-faceted approach which minimizes use of pharmaceuticals and surgery and instead emphasizes the use of harmless lifestyle and dietary changes, plus vitamins, minerals and herbal supplements.

Hypothyroidism or **Low Thyroid Condition.** A common cause of chronic tiredness resulting from a sluggish thyroid gland which slows the body's entire metabolism and often leads to weight increase. Hypothyroidism is most common in women. (See "Hypothyroidism—Low Thyroid Condition" in Chapter 2.)

Insulin. A hormone released by the pancreas to normalize the body's blood sugar level. Insulin lowers the blood sugar level by converting surplus glucose into glycogen for storage in the liver and muscles.

Iron-Deficiency Anemia. A common cause of chronic tiredness in women (and sometimes in men), iron-deficiency anemia results from a loss of blood which leads to an iron deficiency. Without sufficient iron, the bloodstream is unable to transport oxygen to body cells and the result is chronic fatigue. (See "Iron-Deficiency Anemia" in Chapter 2.)

Krebs Cycle. The series of biochemical reactions through which our bodies metabolize carbohydrates into energy to fuel the muscles.

Low Blood Sugar or **Hypoglycemia.** When large amounts of refined carbohydrates are consumed, glucose floods into the bloodstream, overwhelming the ability of the pancreas to secrete insulin and to store surplus glucose as glycogen in the muscles and liver. However, the surplus glucose is soon used up and without glycogen reserves to draw on, the blood sugar level plummets. The result is Low Blood Sugar, which is the same as feeling drained of energy.

Mini-Meals. Dividing three regular-sized daily meals into six or nine smaller portions or mini-meals and eating them at regular intervals throughout the day. The total amount of food consumed in mini-meals never exceeds the total normally eaten in three conventional meals.

Nocturnal Myoclonus. Also called Periodic Leg Movement, Nocturnal Myoclonus is a sleep-disturbing disease which almost invariably leads to chronic tiredness.

Nonheme. One of two forms of dietary iron, nonheme exists in plant foods. Only three percent of iron in plant foods can normally be absorbed by humans.

Paradoxical Intent. Based on behavioral psychology, Paradoxical Intent helps you to achieve a goal by having you try to do exactly the opposite. For example, if you are in bed and cannot sleep, try to stay awake instead. The odds are you will swiftly fall asleep. (See FF#16.)

Passive Therapy. A treatment in which something is given you, or done to you, by someone else and you play only a passive role in your own recovery. Among passive therapies are drugs, surgery, massage and herbal medicines prescribed by others.

Positive Thinking. The brainchild of Dr. Norman Vincent Peale, Positive Thinking changes the way people feel by changing the way they think. Allowing only positive thoughts in the mind ensures that you experience only positive, upbeat feelings.

Postprandial Dip. An energy slump that occurs around 3:00 p.m. in people who eat a heavy lunch high in fat or fried foods or refined carbohydrates. (See under "Energy Booster #8" in FF#11-A.)

Preventive Medicine. That branch of medicine concerned with learning how to live a healthy, active life while remaining free of the same chronic diseases that mainstream medicine endeavors to treat.

Protein. The stuff of which muscles, bones, cartilage, skin, blood, enzymes, hormones and antibodies are formed, protein is essential for the growth, repair and maintenance of the body. But whether of vegetable or animal origin, it is a poor source of energy for fueling muscles.

Relaxation Response. The opposite of the Fight or Flight Response, the Relaxation Response is a state in which mind and body are both calm and relaxed. When a person is in the Relaxation Response, muscular tension and mental anxiety and depression fade away and the entire bodymind remains in a state of optimal health.

Slow-Twitch Muscles. These muscles, used in aerobic exercise, respond slowly to the challenge of exercise but once moving rhythmically, they can keep you going for hours.

Sports Drinks. Bottled drinks for athletes containing glucose polymers, designed to help replace glycogen reserves plus minerals and other nutrients that may be lost in sweat. Most nutritionists consider sports drinks to be non-essential.

Stimulus Control Behavior Therapy. A behavioral approach to overcoming insomnia which allows you to remain in bed only while asleep. (See FF#14.)

Training Effect. A sudden increase in cardiovascular fitness and stamina that occurs in most people after they take up a graduated aerobic exercise program. To achieve training effect, you must walk in your heart target zone range for 20 minutes or longer three to five times each week or more often. Training effect occurs as the body maximizes its oxygen uptake. It can be achieved through any type of rhythmic aerobic exercise.

Warm-Up. Warming up the muscles before exercising by taking a short, moderately-paced walk (or other rhythmic exercise) and then stretching the now-warm muscles. Warming-up prevents joint and muscle injury and also stimulates the liver to begin releasing glycogen to fuel the muscles during the upcoming exercise.

BIBLIOGRAPHY

Ahlquist, J. E.; Sibley, C. G. "Phylogeny of the Hominoid Primates as Indicated by DNA-DNA Hybridization." *Journal of Molecular Evolution*, 20, 1984; pp 2-15.

Anderson, Owen. "Mind Over Matter." *Runner's World*, May 1992, p 26.

Applegate, Liz. "Nutrition: Give It a Rest." *Runner's World*, October 1991, pp 22-24. "Nutrition: Good Solutions (sports drinks)." *Runner's World*, July 1992, pp 18-21.

Baird, Pat. *Quick Harvest: A Vegetarian's Guide to Microwave Cooking*. Prentice Hall, 1991.

Barnard, Neal D., M.D. *The Power Of Your Plate*. Book Publishing Company, 1990.

Borysenko, Joan, Ph.D. *Minding The Body, Mending The Mind*. Addison-Wesley, 1987.

Burke, Susan G. "Chronic Fatigue Syndrome and Women: Can Therapy Help?" *Social Work*, January 1992, pp 35-39.

Burns, David, M.D. *Feeling Good Handbook*. NAL-Dutton, 1990. *Feeling Good: The New Mood Therapy*. Avon, 1992.

Chaitow, Leon. *The Beat Fatigue Workbook: How to Identify*

the Cause and Discover New Vitality. Thorsons SF (U.K.), 1989.

Chauner, Walt. "Ski Better With Age," *Skiing*, February 1992, pp 62-63.

Chopra, Deepak M.D. *Quantum Healing: Exploring the Frontiers of Bodymind Medicine.* Bantam, 1990.

Cox, I.; Campbell, J.; et al. "Red Blood Cell Magnesium and Chronic Fatigue Syndrome." *Lancet*, 1991: 337, pp 757-760.

Dell Medical Library Staff. *Learning to Live With Chronic Fatigue Syndrome.* Dell, 1990.

"Depression." *Public Citizen Health Letter*, April 1989, pp 1-6.

Diamond, Jared. "Dawn of the Human Race." *Discover*, May 1989.

Eaton, S. Boyd., M.D.; Konner, Melvin J., M.D., Ph.D.; Shostak, Marjorie. "Stone Agers in the Fast Lane: Chronic and Degenerative Diseases in Evolutionary Perspective." *American Journal of Medicine*, 84, 1988; pp 735-747.; *The Paleolithic Prescription*, Harper & Row, 1989.

Ebbert, Stephanie. "Fight Off Chronic Fatigue." *Prevention*, January 1991, pp 33-43.

Faelton, Sharon; Diamond, David and the Editors of *Prevention* Magazine. *Take Control of Your Life.* Rodale Press, 1988.

Feiden, Karyn. *Hope and Help For Chronic Fatigue Syndrome: the Official Book of the CPS—CFIDS Network.* Prentice Hall, 1990.

Ford, Norman D. *Good Health Without Drugs.* St. Martin's Press, 1979; *Natural Ways to Relieve Pain.* Harian Press, 1980; *Minding Your Body.* Autumn Press, 1981; *Arthritis and Gout.* Prentice Hall, 1982; *Goodnight to*

Insomnia. Para Research, 1983; *Sleep Well, Live Well.* Zebra Books, 1984; *Lifestyle for Longevity.* Para Research, 1985; *Formula For Long Life*, Harian Press, 1986; *Eighteen Natural Ways to Beat The Common Cold.* Keats Publishing, 1987; *Eighteen Natural Ways to Beat a Headache.* Keats Publishing, 1988; *Keep on Pedaling.* Countryman Press, 1990; *The Healthiest Places to Live and Retire*, Ballantine Books, 1992; *Walk to Your Heart's Content.* Countryman Press, 1992; *Eighteen Natural Ways to Lower Your Cholesterol.* Keats Publishing, 1992.

Franklin, Mike; Sullivan, Jane. *The New Mystery Fatigue Epidemic.* Century (U.K.) Trafalgar, 1990.

Gardner, David C.; Beatty, Grace J. *Never Be Tired Again.* Harper Collins, 1990.

Garfield, Charles A., *Peak Performance.* Warner Books, 1989.

Gawain, Shakti. *Creative Visualization.* Bantam, 1983.

Geiger, Lura J. *Burnout: Renewing Your Energy.* Luramedia, 1987.

Gutfield, Greg. "Beat Chronic Fatigue." *Prevention*, August 1991, pp 8-9.

Hales, Diana. "What's Making Me Tired? How to Escape the No-Energy Trap." *Family Circle*, January 8, 1991, pp 43-44.

Hauri, Peter; Linde, Shirley. *No More Sleepless Nights.* Wiley Books, 1991.

Heimlich, Jane. *What Your Doctor Won't Tell You.* Harper Collins, 1990.

Hittleman, Richard. *Richard Hittleman's 28-Day Yoga Exercise Plan.* Workman Publishing, 1969.

Inlander, Charles B.; Lowell, S. Levin. *Medicine on Trial.* Prentice Hall, 1988.

Jampolsky, Gerald G., M.D. *Love is Letting Go of Fear.*

Bantam, 1981; *Goodbye to Guilt*. Bantam, 1985; *Out of Darkness into Light*. Bantam, 1989.

Katzenstein, Larry et al. "Sick and Tired." *American Health*, May 1992, pp 51-56.

Kaufman, Wallace. "Virus Hunter—Chronic Fatigue Syndrome." *American Health*, May 1992, pp 33-35.

Kendell, R.E. "Chronic Fatigue, Viruses and Depression." *Lancet*, January 19, 1991, pp 160-162.

Keyes, Ken. *Handbook to Higher Consciousness*. Love Line Books, 1975.

Krakovitz, Rob, M.D. *High Energy*. Jeremy Tarcher, Inc., 1986.

Lappé, Frances Moore. *Diet For a Small Planet*. Ballantine Books, 1982.

Layzer, Robert B. "How Muscles Use Fuel." *New England Journal of Medicine*, Vol. 324, February 7 1991, pp 411-412.

Levin, Susanne. "The Burnout Factor." *Women's Sports & Fitness*, August 1991, pp 12-13.

Lewinsohn, Peter M., et al. *The Coping With Depression Course*. Castalia Publishers, 1984.

Lutter, Jody Mahle. "The Strength-Sapping Sickness." *Women's Sports & Fitness*, October 1991, pp 22-24.

McDougall, John, M.D. *The McDougall Plan*. New American Library, 1991.

McQuade, Molly. "Fifty Things You Should Know About Chronic Fatigue Syndrome." *Publishers Weekly*, April 27 1992, p 265.

Martorano, Joseph T.; Kildahl, John P. *Beyond Negative Thinking*. Insight Books, 1989.

Mehta, Silva, et al. *Yoga: the Iyengar Way*. Knopf, 1990.

Nolan, Donna D. *Ending Fatigue and Depression*. James & McCormick, Publishers, 1988.

Parkes, J. D. *Sleep and Its Disorders.* Saunders Books, 1986.

Peale, Norman Vincent. *You Can If You Think You Can.* Prentice Hall, 1987. *Power of Positive Thinking Book.* Fawcett, 1992. *Six Attitudes For Winners.* Tyndale Books, 1990.

Podell, Richard N. *Doctor, Why Am I So Tired?* Pharos Books, 1988.

Pritikin, Robert. *The New Pritikin Program.* Simon & Schuster, 1991.

Rubinbach, Anson. *The Human Motor: Energy, Fatigue and Origins of Modernity.* Basic Books, 1990.

Reisser, Paul. *Energy Drainers, Energy Gainers.* Zondervan Books, 1990.

Rosenthal, Norman E. *Seasons of the Mind.* Bantam, 1990.

Ross, Harvey M.; Roth, June. *Mood Control Diet: Twenty-One Days to Conquering Depression and Fatigue.* Prentice Hall, 1990.

Selby, John. *Secrets Of a Good Night's Sleep.* Avon Books, 1989.

Sheehan, George. "Athletic Wisdom." *Runner's World,* January 1992, p 14.

Smidt, Laurie J., et al. "Influence of Thiamine Supplementation on the Health and General Well-Being of an Elderly Irish Population with Marginal Thiamine Deficiency." *Journals of Gerontology,* January 1990, pp M16-M22.

Strickland, Bill. "What's Wrong With This Breakfast?" *Bicycling,* October 1992, p 72.

Sweeny, Donald R. *Overcoming Insomnia.* Bantam, 1991.

Troiano, Linda R. "The Better Way: Tired All The Time? You Could Have CFS!" *Good Housekeeping,* January 1991, pp 165-166.

Underwood, Nora. "Sick and Tired." *Macleans,* February 4, 1991, p. 52.

Van Gelder, Lindsy. "Women and Anemia: Are You Iron-Deficient or Just Worn out?" *Glamour*, December 1991, pp 50-52.

Wasco, James. "Your Body, Your Health: When Vague Symptoms Are Dangerous." *Woman's Day*, March 5 1991, p 18.

Woods, B.; Martin, L.; Andrew, P. *Major Topics in Primate and Human Evolution*. Cambridge University Press, 1986.

Zinchenko, Vladimir. *The Psychometrics of Fatigue*. Taylor & Francis, 1984.

INDEX

249

ABOUT THE AUTHOR

Norman D. Ford is a medical researcher and reporter, a self-help author and an expert in natural and holistic therapies. He has written for *Prevention, Woman's Day* and other well-known health-oriented magazines and has lectured extensively to health groups and organizations. Ford has authored more than 50 books in the fields of retirement, leisure and health. He practices what he preaches and his lifestyle is built on the same Whole-Person health practices described in this book. At age 72, Ford has an abundance of energy and he remains an avid hiker, bicyclist, swimmer and vegetarian and has practiced yoga regularly for many years. He lives in the Hill Country of Texas and frequently hikes and mountain-bicycles in Colorado and Utah.